To Lu

"Sleep Well"

"Danny"

Mark J____ (, MD)

Deadly — — Sleep

Is Your Sleep Killing You?

A Common Sleep Disorder
Could Be Destroying you!

How You Can Save Your Life and the
Lives of Your Loved Ones

Mack D. Jones, MD

iUniverse, Inc.
New York   Bloomington

Deadly Sleep
Is Your Sleep Killing You?

iUniverse books may be ordered through booksellers or by contacting:

iUniverse
1663 Liberty Drive
Bloomington, IN 47403
www.iuniverse.com
1-800-Authors (1-800-288-4677)

ISBN: 978-0-595-52870-7 (pbk)
ISBN: 978-0-595-62925-1 (ebk)

Printed in the United States of America

iUniverse rev. date: 8/17/2009

Front cover: MRI-DTI brain scan of one of 41 men and women, ages 38 to 52,
with obstructive sleep apnea and multiple strokes; "Brain Structural Changes in
Obstructive Sleep Apnea," by Paul M Macey, et al. SLEEP 2008; 31(7): 967-977.

Dedication ——————————————

I DEDICATE THIS BOOK to the memory of my father, Henry Madison "Mack" Jones, who died in 1998 from complications of Alzheimer's disease, a consequence of sleep apnea.

Contents

Acknowledgments ━━━━━━

I WOULD LIKE TO thank those who shared their personal experiences of sleep apnea with me. Their tragic stories and many questions were the stimulus for this book.

A special thanks to Mary Lou Kruger, Jackie Youngblood, and Lynn Bowling for their invaluable assistance and moral support.

Introduction ━━━━━━━━━━━━━

Ten years ago, I made the decision to take on sleep disorders medicine as a subspecialty in my field of neurology. Within two years, I discovered I had sleep apnea (SA) myself and began my search for a cure. After surviving the four-year ordeal, I decided to put into writing the discoveries I made, to answer questions for patients who were struggling with signs and symptoms of sleep apnea.

The focus here is on sleep apnea, specifically, obstructive sleep apnea (OSA), which is the single-most common problem seen by sleep specialists today. It is also very poorly understood, not only by the general public but by many in the medical community as well.

As a clinical neurologist with a special interest in sleep disorders prior to being diagnosed with SA, I have a unique perspective that could be of value to anyone with questions about the disorder.

The purpose of this book is to wake up the reader to a serious problem in our society—a problem, I suspect, that has been with us for hundreds if not thousands of years.

I aim it at the layperson, or nonmedical reader, so they might better understand the problems of SA. Some of what I have to say is controversial and open to different interpretations, because within the past ten years that I have studied this condition and as a former OSA patient myself, I have developed an undeniably different point of view regarding some aspects of this most deadly disease.

There are several excellent sources of more detailed information available on the Internet, in bookstores, and in libraries in which you can find answers to questions that may not have been addressed here (see Appendix B, Further Reading). I would like to caution you, however, that you may encounter what I call "the party line." This is the kind of information that gets into the literature and is accepted and repeated so much so that it almost becomes a mantra. No one questions it until someone stands up and says, "Wait a minute, this doesn't apply anymore. You are not keeping up with the current technology."

I will touch on some of these issues, for example, the continued insistence on prescribing the continuous positive airway pressure (CPAP) machine instead of the more advanced Autotitrating PAP (APAP) machine or the continued practice of performing certain surgical procedures when they are of questionable benefit.

I recommend you look at several sources. From different points of view, you may see problems that have not been fully addressed, or you may even recognize contradictory statements and start asking your own questions.

In addition to discussing the basics, I will emphasize an area that has been overlooked or outright ignored: that OSA is not only a likely cause of Alzheimer's disease (AD)—a stunning revelation in itself—but also a potential cause or major contributor to a host of other life-threatening diseases and disorders that have been with us for a very long time. The untold story of OSA and its consequences are, to put it mildly, mind-boggling.

OSA affects every part of our society to a degree that is almost incomprehensible. An estimated 18 million Americans have sleep apnea. Millions more are predisposed and have a high risk of developing the illness. Many victims have no symptoms, or relatively minor ones, for many years until the symptoms finally become obvious as recognizable signs of the disease. Who out there has the disorder? How do you detect it? And what can you do about it once it is diagnosed? Here, in this book, are my answers to these questions presented in six chapters. Real-life examples are included in case histories at the end of the book. I have included a few Web sites and books that I have found informative for those who desire to pursue the subject in more detail.

I began writing this with the sleep apneic reader in mind, with two major goals: to alert the public to this life-threatening disorder and to prompt those who get the message into action on their own behalf or on behalf of a loved one.

I have been there, so to speak, and have come back to tell my story. Viewing SA from the inside out is not the preferred means of learning about the disorder, but the experience led me to some surprising realizations. I will explain, with as little medical jargon as possible, what I discovered and what it takes to avoid some of the pitfalls I encountered before finally conquering this scourge of the night: sleep apnea.

Chapter 1. ━━━━━━━━━━━━━
What Is Sleep Apnea?

THERE ARE THREE MAJOR types of sleep apnea (SA), determined by an overnight sleep test:

1. Obstructive sleep apnea (OSA), repeated airway obstructions during sleep. It is the most common type (84 percent of the sleep apnea population) and the major topic of discussion in this book.
2. Central sleep apnea (CSA), nerve cells in the brain stem fail to trigger automatic breathing (uncommon, at less than 1 percent).
3. Complex sleep apnea syndrome (CSAS), a combination of the two above (15 percent).

Obstructive Sleep Apnea

During sleep, relaxed soft tissues and muscles in the back of the throat just behind the tongue (and sometimes the tongue itself) are sucked into the upper airway by the vacuum created when inhaling, blocking the flow of air down into the lungs. This airway blockage, or obstruction of airflow, is called "apnea" (pronounced "AP-nee-yuh"), from Greek, meaning "breathless, or no breath." These obstructive

1

apneas may last from several seconds to minutes and occur repeatedly while asleep.

In the typical patient, apneas occur night after night, year after year. They may extend throughout most of one's adult life and, in some cases, throughout one's entire lifetime.

Symptoms of Obstructive Sleep Apnea

One or more of the following symptoms may occur:

- Unrefreshed sleep
- Snoring (80 percent of OSA patients snore)
- Excessive daytime sleepiness or drowsiness
- Insomnia, waking up and having difficulty going back to sleep
- Hyper-arousal or sense of heightened awareness, feeling "wired"
- Early morning headache or chronic headache
- Suddenly waking up gasping, choking, or snorting
- Waking up with a sense of drowning
- Waking up hot or sweaty
- Waking with a dry mouth or sore throat
- Fatigue, tiredness, physical exhaustion
- Unexplained weight gain or difficulty losing weight
- Heartburn or gastroesophageal reflux disease (GERD)
- Frequently getting up at night to urinate
- Reduced libido
- Clumsiness, poor coordination
- Bed wetting
- Irritability, mood swings, personality change
- Anger, frustration, road rage, and such behaviors
- Confusion
- Job burnout
- Sports skills decline
- Poor decision making
- Forgetfulness

- Depression
- Inability to concentrate
- Sleepwalking
- Or no symptoms at all...yet!

Note: Denial of symptoms is common in patients with known SA. It is my contention that most victims either have no symptoms early on, or have minor symptoms attributed to or passed off as being due to some unrelated condition; they are unaware that OSA is the actual underlying cause. This can go on for years before the first clear symptom appears. Dr. William Dement, considered the "father of sleep medicine," has said, "It is possible for individuals to be entirely normal awake and deadly ill asleep."

The first indication of OSA may be a major complication, such as obesity, high blood pressure, diabetes, heart attack, stroke, or other serious illness (see lists in Chapter 2).

Holding one's breath voluntarily is not the same as an obstruction of the airway during sleep. When we can no longer hold our breath, we simply let go and start breathing again, but when we are asleep and cannot breathe, the brain recognizes this as a life-threatening emergency and the alarms go off.

When an apnea occurs in sleep, there are at least three major problems that strike like a shot from an imaginary "triple-barreled shotgun," blasting away at every living cell in the body. First, there is a drop in blood oxygen (hypoxia), measured with a pulse oximeter attached to a finger or earlobe (normal blood oxygen level is greater than 95 percent). Hypoxia may be mild to severe, with blood oxygen levels falling to 90, 80, 70 percent, or lower. There is an accompanying rise in blood carbon dioxide (CO_2). I'll describe what this does to the heart and brain in a moment.

Second is an emergency stress reaction (sympathetic nervous system stimulation), in which there is a sudden surge in stress hormones, many from the adrenal glands (cortisol, adrenaline, epinephrine, etc.) and others from the brain, as part of the sympathetic nervous system's emergency "fight or flight" mechanism. Blood pressure rises, heart rate and breathing rate increase, and profuse sweating may occur—it's as if a grizzly bear were chasing you and you were running for your life!

This reaction is in part responsible for the damage to the cells that line the inner walls of arteries, causing atherosclerosis and leading to high blood pressure, heart attack, sudden cardiac death, stroke, and so on.

There is a significant suppression of the immune system accompanied by signs of chronic inflammation, which leaves the body defenseless against invasive viruses, bacteria, or foreign proteins, resulting, potentially, in a multitude of diseases.

Third is the problem of sleep deprivation or sleep debt. Sleep disruptions destroy normal restorative cycles, resulting in mild to severe sleep debt. If sleep deprivation can kill animals under experimental conditions, it cannot be good for us.

The brain requires a full night's uninterrupted sleep to function optimally. Anything less and it begins to fail us. During sound sleep, our priceless, three-pound neurobiological supercomputers consolidate memories; are restored, recharged, and refreshed; undergo new cell growth (neurogenesis); and are returned to a normal functional state. Our adult brains require about seven to eight hours of sound sleep to do this. A good night's sleep can be the difference between acing an exam and flunking it. We are reminded daily of the consequences of sleep deprivation from the unending carnage resulting from motor vehicle crashes. It is responsible for 100,000 police-reported motor vehicle accidents, over 175,000 injuries, and at least 1,550 deaths yearly.

Any one of these three conditions (chronic low blood oxygen, repeated stress reactions, and years of sleep deprivation) occurring independently can be devastating. The three occurring together, as in OSA, are catastrophic.

How Do You Diagnose OSA?

In most cases, the diagnosis is confirmed by performing an overnight sleep test or polysomnogram (PSG) in an accredited sleep laboratory. The patient sleeps in a quiet, comfortable, temperature-controlled room, similar to a motel room. Several monitors are connected by placing leads on the scalp, face, chest, arms, and legs and are reviewed on a video screen by a registered technician in a separate control room. An infrared video camera records any movements or atypical activity. The technician is able to visualize the heart rate, blood oxygen, breathing pattern, brain waves (via electroencephalogram, or EEG), eye movements, and arm and leg movements throughout the night. The test can determine normal versus abnormal sleep.

The diagnosis of sleep apnea can be made by simply observing the person while asleep. Loud snoring with frequent long pauses (obstructed breathing) can get the attention of a victim's bed partner, leading to an evaluation by a sleep specialist and successful treatment.

Home testing (HT) or portable monitoring systems are becoming more available now that Medicare has approved payment for their use. Recent studies have shown that home testing is as effective as the in-laboratory PSG for establishing a diagnosis.[1] Many patients have difficulty sleeping in the laboratory and do much better in their own beds at home in familiar surroundings.

The inability to sleep in the lab is called the "First night effect." The patient lies awake all night, uncomfortable in this unfamiliar environment. Some of these patients are misdiagnosed because an inexperienced or inadequately trained tech misinterprets the brain waves on the video monitor thinking the patient is asleep when he is actually wide awake. Ten percent of the normal population has brain waves that have the appearance of light sleep when they are awake with their eyes closed. The patient can be misdiagnosed "normal" when he never went to sleep. This is one reason for a "false negative" test which has been shown to occur in up to 15 to 25 percent of cases in some accredited sleep labs.

Dr. Barbara Phillips, MD, MSPH, a past president of the National Sleep Foundation (NSF), has made the point, with supportive evidence,[2,3] that one apnea per hour can be "deadly," and therefore, all obstructions must be eliminated. This message has been slow to get out into the medical community.

The apnea-hypopnea index (AHI) is used to indicate the average number of apneas and hypopneas (shallow breathing) that occur per hour throughout a night's sleep. The degree of severity is classified as mild (five to fourteen per hour), moderate (fifteen to thirty per hour), and severe (greater than thirty per hour). Note: Fewer than five per hour, in adults, is considered "normal" or "acceptable" in the world of sleep medicine (I have some difficulty with that, when only one obstruction per hour can be deadly, as stressed by Dr Phillips). One apnea per hour is eight per night, or 2,920 per year. In seventy years, you have 204,400 obstructions. Is that enough to cause adverse consequences? Potentially yes, because what must be taken into account is how prolonged the apneas are, how severe the drops in blood oxygen levels are and how the apneas are distributed throughout the night? For example, are they occurring mostly during the latter part of the night, when rapid eye movement (REM) sleep predominates? There is presumably greater risk if apneas are grouped together rather than spread out evenly throughout the night. Remember, the AHI is the total number of apneas and hypopneas divided by the number of hours of sleep. The severity of any one or combination of these factors can make a significant difference in the overall outcome over a period of many years.

The adverse effects of each apnea are additive or cumulative, a dynamic and highly variable process that will likely catch up with you eventually.

Get out your calculator and check the numbers of potential apneas in a more realistic setting, and you will wonder how some apneics manage as well as they do. The infant or young child's rapidly developing brain is considerably more vulnerable and doesn't stand a chance against undetected OSA. (An AHI of 1 is abnormal in children).

Sleep apnea is common. There are an estimated 18 million Americans with it in the general population (20 percent of men and 9 percent of women between thirty and sixty years old in one large study[4]).

In a study of a group seventy years old and older, 76 percent of men and 54 percent of women had OSA. It is estimated that 80 to 90 percent of victims are undiagnosed, and the majority of those are asymptomatic. My bet is that OSA is considerably more common throughout the United States and the world than is generally thought and is probably pandemic. (A pandemic is a widespread epidemic that may affect entire continents or even the world).

Sleep apnea is deadly. Repeated apneas over many years can kill you; therefore, all obstructions must be prevented. Reggie White, NFL Hall of Famer, and Jerry Garcia, Grateful Dead guitarist, come to mind. Both were thought to have died from complications of SA. There are many others.

SA is chronic and progressively gets worse with age and weight gain. It affects all age groups and is estimated to be found in about 9 percent of Caucasians, 15 to 16 percent of Hispanics and African Americans, and 24 percent of Asians. You may be surprised to read that Asians have a higher incidence as I was when I first read it. The explanation is that Asians have anatomically small upper airways as part of their genetic makeup.

Apneas are generally worse when sleeping on your back (the tongue falls back into the airway) and less severe sleeping on your side (the tongue falls to one side). Some patients have apneas only when sleeping on their backs and have none when sleeping on their sides. But this is subject to change because the airway opening behind the tongue is known to be very dynamic and constantly changing with age, weight gain or loss, allergies, and upper respiratory infections, so that you cannot depend on the airway remaining the same.

This unpredictability of the size of the airway can present problems with long-term treatment. I'll discuss this further in Chapter 3.

Tennis balls sewn into the back of a nightshirt have been recommended for years as a means of staying off one's back while asleep. The idea seemed to be a good one (I recommended it many times for patients during my practice), but it turns out that many patients ignore the tennis balls and continue to sleep on their backs anyway. I had the same experience myself when I tried it several years ago. Some newer vest like devices with large humps on the back may be more successful by making it physically impossible to sleep on your back.

All snoring is abnormal until proven otherwise. Approximately 70 percent of snorers have SA. Eighty percent of SA patients snore, most loudly, some softly. I suspect that many if not most snorers who don't have SA now, will eventually develop it.

Sleep apnea is not taken seriously, even by most in the medical profession. How many doctors ask you or your spouse about your sleep?

Sleep apnea is a medical urgency—in some, it is an emergency. How many apneas or obstructions are you having while you wait for your referral to a sleep specialist, wait for your sleep test, wait for your CPAP titration, wait for your next appointment, wait for your surgery, or wait to heal after one surgery before the next surgery? In my opinion, waiting (piling up the apneas) can be very bad for your health. Let's stop piling up the apneas!

Chapter 2. ——
The Consequences

Brain Structural Changes in Obstructive Sleep Apnea

A NUMBER OF NEUROIMAGING studies have been performed on patients with OSA including CT, MRI, PET, and single photon emission computed tomography (SPECT) scans, revealing various defects, but none has displayed anything quite as astonishing or as dramatic as the study published in *SLEEP* July 1, 2008, by Paul M. Macey et al.[5] The report revealed results of a new MRI technique called diffusion tensor imaging (DTI). Without going into details of this new test, let me tell you that it is an extremely sensitive method of determining damaged nerve fibers (axons) in the brain's white matter. This test, not available until recently, reveals multiple areas of brain damage in OSA patients never known to exist, see an example pictured on the cover.

DTI revealed various sized color-coded yellow-orange patches of brain damage scattered throughout the brains of a group of forty-one men and women with OSA. Their ages ranged from thirty-eight to fifty-two years old, and they had not yet been treated. The areas of nerve fiber injury were located in critical regions of brain including prefrontal, temporal, and parietal lobes. The cerebellum and brainstem were equally involved. This is the first report, to my knowledge, of DTI imaging of a group with OSA. The findings are momentous.

One can anticipate even more areas of damage in older populations when more studies are done. At what age do these brain-damaged areas begin to appear? What problems result from each one of these areas of brain damage? Is it possible that they are responsible for difficulties with cognition, mood, behavior, memory, heart regulation, high blood pressure, breathing control, fear, anxiety, and other emotional disorders, including depression? Could any of these lesions be responsible for fibromyalgia or attention deficit disorder/attention deficit hyperactivity disorder (ADD/ADHD), or eventually accumulate enough to cause Alzheimer's disease? It is fair to say, the possibilities are staggering. The structural changes likely represent accumulated damage over sustained periods. Are they permanent, or do they improve or disappear with treatment? No one knows yet, but my guess is yes, the lesions may improve to some degree or even resolve with treatment, but we will have to wait and see.

The implications of these findings are profound. Early treatment of OSA could potentially prevent the development of Alzheimer's disease. Now is the time to wake up the public and our snoozing medical community and put an end to this disease.

Having obstructive sleep apnea not only is devastating to one's brain and one's health, it can be quite costly, according to the results of a new study.[6] Researchers from Israel found that in the two-year period before diagnosis, health care costs were nearly twice as high for those with OSA compared with those without.

Sleep apnea is a likely cause of many diseases and disorders, some currently acknowledged (Table 1), but many not yet known (Table 2) to the medical community.

Table 1.
Diseases, Disorders, or Conditions That Have a Known Association with OSA

- Accidental death (including auto accidents)
- Ankylosing spondylitis, an inflammatory arthritis with a strong genetic component.
- Cardiac arrhythmias (irregular heartbeat; 50 percent of patients with atrial fibrillation have OSA) Death from sudden cardiac arrest (increased risk during sleep) Heart attack (increased risk during sleep)[7]. Heart risk increases while flying.
- Coronary artery disease (30 to 50 percent of coronary patients have OSA)
- Diabetes, Type 2 (50 percent of people with diabetes have OSA; increased risk of mild cognitive impairment (MCI), which is a risk for Alzheimer's disease or one of the other dementias.
- Depression
- Erectile dysfunction (ED)
- Failed careers (and failed marriages)
- Failure to grow and gain weight (in children)
- Gastroesophageal reflux disease (GERD) increased negative pressures in the chest caused by inhaling through a narrowed upper airway (upper airway resistance), draws or sucks stomach contents into the esophagus and sometimes as far up as the mouth, causing throat, ear, nose and dental complications.
- Headache (tension, migraine, cluster)
- Heart failure (50 percent of people with congestive heart failure have OSA)
- High blood pressure (35 percent of people with high blood pressure have OSA; OSA causes 80 percent of drug-resistant high blood pressure cases)
- Large belly, obesity (77 percent of obese people have OSA; the

incidence of OSA increases with weight gain, as does the risk of mild cognitive impairment)

- Liver disease (non-alcoholic fatty liver disease, or NAFLD; 51 percent of patients with NAFLD have OSA; 50 percent of patients with OSA have NAFLD)
- Pacemakers (59 percent of patients who need pacemakers have OSA)
- Sleepwalking
- Stroke
- Workplace accidents (falling asleep at work while driving a car, truck, or bus; flying an airplane; piloting a ship; operating a train, tending a nuclear reactor, etc.)
- And who knows what else?

Table 2.
Diseases, Disorders, or Conditions That May Be Caused by OSA

Are there diseases with predisposing factors, such as abnormal genes, in which OSA may decrease the threshold for their onset? I think it is highly likely that OSA can be so injurious that it can trigger the onset of some diseases that may not have developed otherwise.

The following conditions have not been studied enough to know how strong the correlations are, if any. Until then, they remain suspect or, in some cases, highly suspect (as, for example, in Alzheimer's disease and in some cases of ADD/ADHD) until proven otherwise by appropriate studies. If this partial list serves no other purpose than to stimulate interest in patients with these disorders to have their sleep status evaluated, it has accomplished its goal.

- Alzheimer's disease and/or the other dementias.
- Attention deficit disorder/attention deficit hyperactivity disorder
- Autism spectrum disorders
- Autoimmune diseases (more than eighty types)

- Bipolar disorder
- Brain tumors
- Cancers (obesity caused by OSA is a risk factor for cancers of the breast, colon, rectum, esophagus, kidneys, ovaries, pancreas, prostate, and uterus)
- Celiac disease
- Chronic fatigue syndrome
- Diabetes, Type 1
- Drug addictions
- Fibromyalgia
- Gout
- HELLP syndrome, a life-threatening obstetric complication usually considered a variant of pre-eclampsia. Both conditions occur during the later stages of pregnancy, or sometimes after childbirth. HELLP is an abbreviation of the main findings: Hemolytic anemia, Elevated Liver enzymes, and Low Platelet count.
- Preeclampsia, and eclampsia
- Irritable bowel syndrome (IBS)
- Kidney failure
- Multiple sclerosis
- Myalgic encephalitis (ME, a term used in Great Britain for a complex constellation of chronic symptoms without a known cause … until now)
- Narcolepsy
- Obsessive-compulsive disorder (OCD)
- Parkinson's disease
- Periodic limb movements of sleep (PLMS)
- Pernicious anemia
- Postpartum depression
- Premature birth
- PTSD
- Restless legs syndrome (RLS)

- Schizophrenia and other psychiatric illnesses
- Seasonal affective disorder (SAD)
- Seizures
- Sensory, motor, and autonomic neuropathies
- Sensory processing disorder (SPD)
- Sudden infant death syndrome (SIDS)
- Suicide
- Tourette's syndrome
- And how many more could be added to or eliminated from this list in the future?

Some critics will say, "This is ridiculous!" or words to that effect. "You might as well throw in the whole textbook of medicine." I think it is fair to say that chronic untreated OSA adversely influences all diseases in the textbook of medicine to some degree. For that reason alone, a sleep test (PSG or HT) is justified.

However, there should be a higher index of suspicion for diseases that may have a genetic susceptibility or higher risk under unusual or extreme conditions. In my opinion, chronic OSA is such a condition. Cellular injury, particularly nerve cell injury brought on by OSA, is an underlying cause. It is well recognized that OSA triggers a cascade of biological reactions, including increased sympathetic nervous system activity, stress hormones, systemic inflammation, oxidative stress, and metabolic alterations that are potentially harmful to multiple systems throughout the body. It is a serious threat. It is stealthy, chronic, and highly destructive. The victim is not only unaware but also, even when informed, often seemingly incapable of fully grasping its seriousness.

Some would argue that it is an "evil" disorder, in that its effect on the brain tends to render one defenseless or seemingly intellectually incapable of defending oneself against the disorder itself.

Table 2 is a partial list of a few diseases that I believe require closer scrutiny by performing a simple sleep test (taking special precautions to avoid the false negative test, which we now know is all too common)

14

and treating those with OSA. What degree of recovery can one expect, and how long will it take? I expect favorable outcomes, but to what extent, over what period, remains to be seen.

If you or your doctor considers the possibility of underlying OSA in connection with these diseases or disorders and has it ruled out by doing a sleep study, the truth will eventually be known as to whether OSA is ultimately responsible. It is a matter of raising the index of suspicion and looking for potential associations. The child with ADD/ADHD is a good example. The word doesn't seem to have gotten out yet; OSA is a cause of ADD/ADHD until proven otherwise.

Since many OSA victims have no symptoms, there is no way to be certain whether a person has it or not. In my opinion, everyone is a potential victim and has OSA until proven otherwise (I know this may sound ridiculous, but bear with me). Everyone should have a sleep test (yes, I realize it's not practical yet due to the expense, but costs will eventually come down with newer technologies).

Those with OSA should be treated regardless of whether there are symptoms or evidence of disease or not. It makes no sense to hold off treatment until a disease develops (the Medicare way), and then begin treatment. The idea is to avoid the disease in the first place. It's called "preventive medicine."

Is there a living cell in the human body that is not adversely influenced to some degree by repeated bouts of hypoxia, excess stress hormones, or sleep deprivation? No, not likely; not a single cell. Show me a disease or disorder that is not potentially made worse by OSA; there is none (even OSA makes itself worse).

Alzheimer's Disease and Other Dementias

Is it possible that obstructive sleep apnea causes Alzheimer's disease or other dementias? I believe so. As a retired clinical neurologist and former OSA patient, I have a special interest in sleep disorders medicine, especially in how it affects the brain and the rest of the nervous system.

I am thoroughly convinced of the connection between OSA and AD, and will remain so until credible studies prove otherwise.

Is the brain capable of withstanding nearly four million apneas extending over a fifty-year period without suffering negative consequences? My answer is no, not likely. Here is a conservative example: A twenty-year-old man has an AHI of 27. That's 27 × 8 hours, or 216 obstructions per night, or 78,840 per year or 3,942,000 apneas by the age of seventy. Of course, in the real world, the numbers of obstructions are subject to considerable variation; in some cases, the number is even greater. The point is that the number of obstructions that any individual may experience during a lifetime are grossly underestimated and take their toll in ways we have failed to recognize.

Numerous short-term studies have been done on cognition (mental processes) and sleep (or the lack thereof), but there are no long-term studies to determine OSA's relationship to Alzheimer's disease or other most common dementias (e.g. Vascular-30 percent, Lewy Body Disease-5 percent, Fronto-Temporal Dementia-5 percent)

At 50–60 percent, Alzheimer's, is the most common of the dementias, affecting an estimated 5.2 million Americans. According to the American Academy of Neurology (ANN), 10 percent of people older than age sixty-five and nearly 50 percent of people older than eighty-five suffer from AD. A 2003 study from *The Archives of Neurology* estimates that there will be 13.2 million Americans with Alzheimer's by the year 2050 if no effective prevention or cure is found.

I have asked experts the question, "Does OSA cause Alzheimer's disease?" And the usual reply is, "No, there is no evidence." There is no evidence because there are no studies directly addressing the issue! Why are there no studies to prove or disprove this question? I cannot answer that, but I suspect there are many reasons, not the least of which is the fragmentation of health specialties into their separate niches with a narrow focus that excludes disorders in the periphery of their specialized fields. The disorder may get lost in the shuffle, so to speak. The lack of financial support is always a big issue. Then, there is reluctance to accept new ideas in direct conflict with long-held beliefs.

Could it be that if OSA proves to be a cause of AD, drugs would no longer be needed? It is almost certain that drugs currently being used would no longer be necessary. The best-case scenario is that AD would rapidly disappear and become a disease of the past. The PAP machine business would certainly do well until something better comes along.

Many polysomnograms (PSGs) have been done on patients with AD, revealing an incidence of OSA of up to 90 percent. The assumption has been that AD causes OSA, or they just happened to coincide, but it is my contention that OSA is a cause if not the cause of AD.

Studies have not been done to address my hypothesis that long-standing undiagnosed OSA is a cause of AD (or one of the other dementias), but evidence is accumulating. For example, OSA is a recognized risk for Type 2 diabetes. In the April 2008 issue of *The Archives of Neurology*, people with Type 2 diabetes were found to have an increased risk of developing mild cognitive impairment[8], which is the earliest stage of dementia. The majority of patients with MCI progress to AD at rate of 12 percent per year.

Additionally, OSA is a known risk for the development of high blood pressure. Like patients with Type 2 diabetes, those with high blood pressure were also found to have an increased risk of developing MCI.[9] Since the majority of patients with MCI eventually progress to Alzheimer's disease at a rate of approximately 12 percent per year, it's not a stretch to conclude that OSA is a cause of Alzheimer's disease. And what about the individual who has both high blood pressure and Type 2 diabetes; is his risk even greater?

A 2006 study in *The Proceedings of the National Academy of Sciences* showed low brain oxygen (hypoxia) raises Alzheimer's risk in the brains of mice with a genetic susceptibility to AD.[10] A group of mice with an Alzheimer's gene were given a maze test in which they all performed normally. They were separated into two groups, one exposed to sixteen hours of a reduced oxygen environment (hypoxia) daily for several weeks; the other group remained in a normal environment.

The maze test was repeated and the hypoxic mice performed poorly, whereas the control group's performance remained normal as before. All the mice were euthanized and their brains examined under a microscope. Plaques and neurofibrillary tangles typical of Alzheimer's disease were present in the hypoxic mouse brain specimens, whereas the controls were normal. According to the investigators, "Hypoxia treatment markedly increased Aβ deposition and neuritic plaque formation and potentiated the memory deficit in Swedish mutant APP transgenic mice. Taken together, our results clearly demonstrate that hypoxia can facilitate AD pathogenesis, and they provide a molecular mechanism linking vascular factors to AD. Our study suggests that interventions to improve cerebral perfusion may benefit AD patients." The study suggests that preventing brain hypoxia (as occurs in OSA) may reduce the risk of developing Alzheimer's disease

Reported in the June 27, 2008 issue of *Neuroscience Letters*, sleep apnea patient were found to have shrunken brain structures called "mammillary bodies" involved in memory, according to Rajesh Kumar and colleagues from the University of California at Los Angeles (UCLA).[11] High-resolution MRI brain scans revealed mammillary bodies to be 20 percent smaller in patients with sleep apnea than in patients without SA. "These findings are important because patients suffering from memory loss from other symptoms, such as alcoholism or Alzheimer's disease, also show shrunken mammillary bodies," Kumar said in a press release.

A recent study from the University of California at San Diego showed that sleep-disordered breathing, including OSA, is an important risk factor for cognitive impairment in older women.[12]

A study from Stanford University School of Medicine in 2001 found a significant portion of sleep-disordered breathing (mostly OSA) is associated with the epsilon4 in the general population[13]. The ApoE epsilon4 gene is a well-known risk factor for Alzheimer's Disease and cardiovascular disease.

Is it too late for the Alzheimer's patient? It may not be. Recent studies showed CPAP-treated Alzheimer's patients experienced improved sleep and quality of life[14] in addition to reduced daytime sleepiness.[15] CPAP improved cognition by increasing total sleep time in a group of AD patients.[16] Obviously, it would be a monumental task to treat large numbers of AD patients with PAP machines or tracheostomies, but with the prospect of improving or reversing the disorder, the idea of more intensive treatment should be given serious consideration.

Attention Deficit Disorder/Attention Deficit Hyperactivity Disorder

Evidence is strong that OSA is a cause of ADD/ADHD in some individuals based on the dramatic results from tonsillectomies and adenoidectomies (T&As; see case 2 in case histories). It is estimated that up to 50 percent of children with ADD/ADHD have OSA; therefore, all children with ADD/ADHD should be checked for OSA and undergo a T&A if needed. Sleep tests can be bypassed in obvious cases where there is strong clinical evidence of OSA (if parents have witnessed snoring or apneas) or if, on examination, the tonsils and adenoids are obviously enlarged and present a problem. A postoperative PSG is recommended to make certain that OSA has been successfully eliminated.

Fibromyalgia Is a Real Disease!

In a recent study of twenty women with fibromyalgia using a brain imaging technique called SPECT (single photon emission computed tomography), Dr. Eric Guedj of Centre Hospitalo-Universitaire de la Timone, of Marseille, France, indicated that the studies revealed abnormally increased blood flow corresponding to a brain region involved in sensing pain and decreased blood flow within an area involved in emotional responses to pain. These findings reinforce the idea that fibromyalgia is a "real disease." They also reinforce my long-held suspicions that fibromyalgia is the result of brain damage from OSA. PSGs and MRI/DTI scans on this group of patients would help settle the question, and successful treatment with PAP should erase all doubts.

Malignant Brain Tumors

Could malignant brain tumors be caused by OSA? Ted Kennedy's recent battle with glioblastoma, the most malignant of brain tumors, received considerable media attention and raised more speculation in the medical community as to the cause. The finding that cytomegalovirus (CMV), a herpes virus, was present in histological specimens has raised the question as to whether the virus itself is responsible. The virus has been considered harmless. Eighty percent of the general population carries the bug. How can this seemingly harmless virus be the cause? It is conceivable that since CMV is not known to attack normal brain cells, it may, however, attack sick or damaged brain cells undergoing repair or regrowth. Older OSA patients have accumulated multiple areas of brain damage,[5] potentially an ideal substrate for an opportunistic virus. Ted Kennedy almost certainly has OSA (given his age, gender, and body profile) and is therefore, at least hypothetically, a candidate for this devastating tumor. Regardless, his presumed OSA must be treated as vigorously as are the other life-threatening problems that he is currently facing.

Chapter 3. ━━━━━━━━━
Treatment

Positive Airway Pressure Machine

THE POSITIVE AIRWAY PRESSURE (PAP) machine is the treatment of choice for adults with OSA. The machine supplies a positive flow of room air through a flexible tube into a mask that fits over the nose or the mouth, acting as a stent to keep the airway open during sleep. This positive airflow prevents the airway from closing. The continuous PAP (CPAP) machine was the original treatment for OSA and continues to be the most frequently prescribed machine for this purpose. With new technologies, it is slowly being replaced by the autotitrating PAP (APAP) machine and, for more complex breathing problems, the ventilator-assisted PAP (VPAP) machine.

The CPAP machine supplies a continuous flow of room air at a predetermined pressure measured in centimeters of water, or cm H_2O (range: 5 to 20-plus cm H_2O, average: 8 to 12 cm H_2O). To be 100 percent effective, the PAP machine must be used 100 percent of sleep-time. When not used during sleep, airway obstructions will occur, defeating the purpose of the machine. If you understand the consequences of treating OSA haphazardly, you will do your best to use your PAP machine faithfully.

Weight loss is equally important in the overweight patient, but while working on weight loss, the PAP machine must be used to reduce the risk of those diseases and disorders listed in Tables 1 and 2.

The mandibular advancement device (MAD) is a custom-fitted mouthpiece made to gradually move the lower jaw (mandible) forward in an attempt to open the back of the throat to eliminate snoring and apneas. It can eliminate snoring, but that is not the real problem. It may reduce the number of apneas, at best, but does not eliminate them altogether; therefore, it should—in my own opinion—be abandoned as a treatment for OSA. I would support its use if it actually worked.

The majority of ear, nose, and throat (ENT) surgeries for OSA in the typical adult at best reduce the AHI, but do not eliminate sleep apnea and should be abandoned. Three exceptions are the following:

1. Tonsillectomy and adenoidectomy (for children with ADD/ADHD).
2. Corrective surgery to make it possible for a patient who is PAP resistant to become PAP successful. An example would be surgical excision of nasal polyps and other conditions that obstruct the nasal airway, allowing some patients to successfully use the PAP machine with the nasal mask.
3. Tracheostomy (the only procedure that can be counted on to cure OSA).

MADs and the majority of ENT surgeries for OSA may reduce the number apneas, but they do not eliminate all apneas (in my case, ENT surgeries actually increased the number of apneas). Note: One apnea or obstruction per hour (apnea-hypopnea index of 1) is "potentially deadly"; therefore, all apneas must be eliminated. If your house is on fire, is it OK for firefighters to leave after putting out only 50 percent or more of the fire? Shouldn't they put out every flame, down to and including the last smoldering ember? Like your house in flames, all obstructive apneas must be extinguished down to and including the last smoldering apnea.

A Dime-Sized Hole in the Neck Beats a Six-Foot Hole in the Ground

If the PAP machines and weight loss fail in spite of maximum effort and there is no likely ENT surgery to convert you from PAP resistance to PAP success, then the final step is a tracheostomy. A small opening in the trachea bypasses the obstructions in the upper airway and eliminates the problem once and for all.

After your tracheostomy has healed, you can, at your leisure (and free of all those apneas for the first time in years), try out any of the surgical procedures offered for OSA, and if one actually eliminates all apneas or converts you to a PAP success, then the tracheostomy can be reversed (surgically closed). I have that option myself, but have no interest in experimenting further with surgeries.

My bias is that under these circumstances, there would be very few patients (if any, like myself) who would proceed to a reversal or closure of their tracheostomy. That is because I do not believe there are presently any ENT procedures capable of reliably eliminating all apneas. Surgical conversion to PAP success is another question altogether and may prove to be a viable option. It is a gamble, with an unknown chance of success, but always an option. It should be noted that with a few exceptions, ENT surgeries for OSA are irreversible.

The bottom line: If you already have any of the diseases or disorders listed in Chapter 2, check for OSA; if you have it, seek treatment (with the help of your sleep physician) as soon as possible. The PAP machine may stop OSA's progression, improve your medical condition, or potentially reverse the disorder. It is worth a serious effort. Furthermore, you must continue the use of the PAP machine to prevent future calamities.

If you are healthy, check for OSA anyway. If you have OSA, but no symptoms yet, treat with the PAP machine (with the help of your sleep physician). You may reduce your risk or prevent the diseases or disorders listed above. OSA should be treated regardless of your health status, good or bad. Does it make sense to wait until you get diabetes, high blood pressure, a stroke, or heart attack before going on the PAP machine?

Had you been on the machine all along, you may have never had any of those problems. Case 4 in case histories is an example of a man who waited too long.

Chapter 4.

Searching for a Cure of Obstructive Sleep Apnea: My Four-Year Odyssey

EIGHT YEARS AGO, IT started around three o'clock in the morning. I would wake up and could not get back to sleep (insomnia). During the day, I experienced profound exhaustion or extreme fatigue. This was much more than the tiredness of sleep deprivation, with which I was familiar after working nights in a hospital over the years. I had difficulty describing it. All I could come up with was, "It's like I had been run over by a truck." Not a Ford 150, mind you, but an eighteen-wheeler—a Mack truck.

I didn't feel sleepy in the slightest, but more like I was "wired" or "hyper-alert." This symptom is presumably the result of the sympathetic nervous system going into overdrive, in which adrenal hormones keep you wide awake. My snoring history was not very remarkable. I had been told that I sometimes snored, but not enough to get much attention.

Even though I was not overweight (BMI of 23), I suspected I had obstructive sleep apnea (OSA). I went to see a sleep specialist and had a sleep test—a polysomnogram (PSG); sure enough, I had it. I had OSA. I was blocking my airway twenty-seven times an hour (AHI of 27). Little did I realize at the time that I'd probably had this disorder for many years, and it finally caught up with me. It had gotten my attention for the very first time.

Continuous Positive Airway Pressure

I was prescribed a CPAP machine. It pumps room air at a measured, fixed pressure through a hose attached to a mask that fits over the nose (nasal mask). I went back to the sleep lab for a second night's sleep to have a "CPAP titration," where the air pressure was adjusted to the best single pressure to maintain an open airway. The pressure is measured in centimeters of water. Mine was in the 10 cm H_2O range.

I used the CPAP machine faithfully, 100 percent, with dogged determination, but experienced not the slightest improvement: none, nada. I felt like I was dying. I tried all the PAP machines exactly as prescribed, with no hint of any benefit. "You have to see a surgeon," I was told.

Now at this stage, I was pretty naive about some of the finer details of sleep disorders, especially the surgical treatment of PAP machine-resistant OSA. Sure, I had been going to American Academy of Neurology (AAN) annual meetings and taking courses on sleep disorders, going to seminars, and reading the literature; I even joined the American Academy of Sleep Medicine (AASM) and absorbed everything I could from their annual meetings. Learning from books and meetings is not enough, though, to get a true sense of what OSA is all about. But mix in first-hand experience, as a patient, and that will do the trick.

After some investigation, I saw a highly recommended ENT physician with sixteen years of experience in the surgical treatment of patients with sleep disorders.

Mandibular Advancement Device

Before surgery, I was given a three-month trial on a mandibular advancement device (MAD); this is like a custom-made sports mouth guard that you wear at night; gradually, over months, it ratchets the bottom part of your jaw forward. There are over a hundred varieties of MADs made. They force the lower jaw and tongue outward or forward and are supposed to open the airway.

After three months of faithfully adjusting this device every other night, I experienced no change—nothing. It just moved my teeth around, making them more crooked than they were already. My opinion of the device? Just thinking about it makes me "MAD." Keep in mind that all the while I am going through this trial-and-error period, I am blocking my airway twenty-seven times an hour. That is twenty-seven times eight hours, times thirty days, times three months = 19,440 obstructions.

ENT Surgeries for OSA

This was followed by an uvulopalatopharyngoplasty (UPPP, or UP3), a procedure where the uvula, part of the soft palate, tonsils, and adenoids are surgically removed. Still no hint of any benefit—nothing.

We also tried a hyoid myotomy (the hyoid muscle is cut loose from the hyoid bone above the Adam's apple). You guessed it. No improvement, nada, zip.

Then, we tried rhinoplasty (three procedures on the nose including straightening the nasal septum). Nothing, no improvement.

Then, we tried another rhinoplasty, a revision; ditto, no improvement.

That is 164,640 more obstructions, a very rough estimation since it is impossible to know precisely, because of the dynamic nature and wide variations in the number of apneas (unless, of course, some kind of continuous monitor is used, which is not yet practical).

Note: There are over two dozen surgical procedures that are available, but I will not list them here since none, with rare exception, accomplish a complete resolution of the problem (i.e., no more obstructions).

Did I say I was getting desperate? I was miserable; I could not think or concentrate. My number one hobby, reading, was no longer pleasurable. I had trouble remembering what I had just read. I was irritable and had an almost constant low-grade headache. What day was it? Once I got lost and took the wrong off-ramp on a trip back to Florida from Atlanta. A sudden fear came over me. I was lost. Finally, I got my bearings and made my way home.

Depressed? No, but upset, angry that I was getting nowhere. As a neurologist, I knew that my thinking abilities had dropped well below par. I had done the mini-mental state examination (MMSE) on many patients during my career, and now I was performing the test, somewhat haphazardly, on myself, and I was not doing very well. I wouldn't have been at all surprised that if I were formally tested, I might have come very close to being classified as having mild cognitive impairment (MCI), or an early dementia.

I was toast.

There is an approximate three- to six-month recovery or healing period between some surgeries. I asked about surgically removing a portion of the back of my tongue, a linguoplasty. My surgeon was reluctant because there is a high risk of post-surgical complications like swelling of the remaining tongue, causing obstruction of the airway immediately after the operation (an elective tracheostomy is usually done before surgery just in case of such an emergency).

Finally, I asked, "How about a tracheostomy?" Its success rate is 99-plus percent. A tracheostomy makes a small opening about the size of the end of your little finger in the trachea below the Adam's apple and just above the notch in the breastbone, or sternum. This procedure is the so-called medical gold standard, i.e., the one procedure that will get rid of the problem once and for all, or cure it. The obstructed airway is simply bypassed, allowing you to breathe freely through an opening in the trachea. The success rate would be 100 percent if it were not for uncommon complications like infection or bleeding (and even death in rare cases reported years ago). These days, the risk is probably no greater than that of most any other surgical procedure done for OSA by an experienced ENT surgeon.

OK, I was scheduled for a tracheostomy early Monday morning. During the weekend before the surgery, my CPAP machine suddenly and dramatically seemed to be working, an experience I had never had. I woke up Saturday and Sunday mornings feeling surprisingly alert and rested. I had adjusted the pressure down to 5 cm H_2O (it had never been that low before), and it seemed to work. I called my surgeon and discussed it with him, and he decided to postpone the tracheostomy until I gave the CPAP machine a little more time. Had I finally found the magic CPAP pressure? It lasted about three to four days, and then it was back to square one—the old "eighteen-wheeler" again.

They repeated the PSG. The only abnormality was a one-hour-and-forty-five-minute period of hypopnea (reduced or shallow breathing, but not complete obstruction) near the middle of the night. I recall remaining awake most of the night; I had what is called "first-night effect." That is when you cannot relax in a strange environment with all the wires stuck to your face and head, chest, arms, and legs, and straps around your chest and abdomen making it cumbersome to turn to get more comfortable—that plus the video camera set up in the corner of the room recording your every move. Without a sleeping pill, it is a miracle that anybody can sleep under those conditions.

I was flummoxed. I was a zombie and my PSG was practically normal except for that short period of hypopnea (and that occurred while I was on my back). I was told to go home and sleep only on my side. That was it. All my sleep problems should have been solved. The only catch—my symptoms continued unchanged.

The only explanation for my lack of improvement that I could come up with was that I could have had undiagnosed upper airway resistance syndrome (UARS).

Upper Airway Resistance Syndrome

I had been to a sleep seminar in St. Petersburg, Florida, where Dr. Christian Guilleminault, a highly respected sleep disorders expert from Stanford University, discussed his concept of a narrowed airway in which one inhales with extra effort (like trying to inhale through a straw), creating a much greater negative pressure in the chest than usual (like -10 to -30 cm H_2O pressure or greater, when normal is -5 cm H_2O pressure).

This, in turn, results in a dramatic change in the flow of blood into and out of the heart, so much so that in some cases the walls of the heart actually collapse. This can cause sudden cardiac death. Dr. Guilleminault showed examples of this with echocardiograms in sleeping patients with UARS. The point was made that the "gold standard" for detecting UARS is an esophageal pressure monitor (Pes monitor). The pressure monitor is attached to the end of a small catheter, passed through the back of the nose, swallowed, and positioned about halfway down the esophagus. It lies in the mid-esophagus during the PSG and measures the negative pressures in the chest as you inhale during the night.

Most sleep techs are not trained to insert these monitors. Patients protest because they can be uncomfortable, and techs do not like to get their patients upset with them even before the test begins. Therefore, most sleep labs do not use them. Instead, they use the unreliable nasal thermistors (heat detectors) for changes in airflow from the nose (more recently, nasal pressure transducers have proven more reliable for this purpose, and most labs are using them).

It took a Pes monitor to test for UARS, and none of the sleep labs in the Southeast routinely used them.

So I made an appointment for a PSG using a Pes monitor at Stanford Sleep Lab, where it was used frequently.

The night of the study, I told the tech that I had had "first-night effect" on two previous PSGs. Without hesitation, she left the room and came back with a sleeping pill (Ambien) to take. Ordinarily, this is a no-no, but in a lab under controlled conditions, it is considered safe.

The reason it is not a good idea to prescribe a sleeping pill to a patient with OSA is that the patient, now sedated, may not arouse as quickly to catch his or her breath, making the apneas more prolonged. This could potentially result in death from cardiac arrest.

This begs the question: How many prescriptions for sleeping pills are written for patients who (unknown to the physician or the patient) have OSA? There may be hundreds of thousands. (My advice: do not use sleeping pills if you do not know whether you have OSA or not.)

Then for the Pes monitor, a couple of swallows of water through a straw, and it was in place. I was surprised at how simple and easy the fifteen-second procedure was. No discomfort whatsoever (this tech should get a raise). I declined the offer for a topical anesthetic to numb the inside of my nose. I could not imagine the need for it. I was awakened once during the night to remove the monitor and went back to sleep for the rest of the night to complete the PSG (and this was the big, bad Pes monitor that all the labs were avoiding, at the patient's peril).

Another question: How many labs using the unreliable heat-sensing airflow monitors (thermistors) miss the diagnosis of UARS and send patients on their way with the erroneous diagnosis of "normal PSG"? Thankfully, the word is out, and most labs no longer rely on the heat-detecting thermistors as their sole means of detecting nasal airflow and UARS. The more reliable nasal pressure transducers are now being used.

The next morning, the attending sleep specialist and his entourage of students, interns, residents, and fellows entered the exam room to discuss the PSG findings (a surreal experience, my being on the receiving end). I had UARS, as I had suspected, but more importantly, I had an AHI of fourty-seven. I have OSA, and I am blocking my airway an average of forty-seven times an hour!

What? Forty-seven! I started with a 27 four years before, tried a MAD; underwent a UPPP, a hyoid myotomy, and two rhinoplasties; and now I am blocking my airway forty-seven times an hour! Another surgery and my AHI might go up to what, sixty-seven? Isn't surgery supposed to make you better? So much for surgery!

Bimax (Maxillomandibular Advancement Surgery)

The recommendation was to undergo more surgery—a bimax or maxillomandibular advancement surgery—because my jaw and airway were congenitally small (it runs in the family). Basically, the jaw (mandible) is sawed loose and moved forward about 10 to 12 mm, and the upper mouth (maxilla) is sawed free and moved forward the same amount. The gaps are filled with bone grafts from the outer layer of the skull or from the pelvis, and there are well-placed pins that hold things in place until healing is complete (six months to a year). Of course, there are potential complications, as with any surgical procedure, but we do not need to go into those details right now.

Hey, I was dying here. Sign me up. The surgery was scheduled for three months (that's forty-seven times eight, times thirty, times three = 33,840 more obstructions until surgery). When I got back home, I dutifully had full dental x-rays and a mold made of my teeth by my dentist. I was to have blood drawn in case I needed it during surgery. I decided to check the bimax surgical literature in a little more detail. I had already read about this surgery, but skimmed over some of the fine print and the disclaimers in several studies, in which their success rates were in the range of 95 percent.

On closer inspection, the word "success" is frequently defined by surgeons as reducing the AHI to less than 20 (still considered "mild sleep apnea") and reducing the total AHI by 50 percent or greater. In my book, if you are stuck with an AHI of anything greater than 0, it is still deadly and cannot be called a "success."

We live in a strange world today, one in which "free" often means "not free" and "success" may just as well mean "not success." Oh, I almost forgot, some years ago some surgeons were using the word "cure" in a similar fashion, but got some criticism for it and decided to switch to "success" instead. I prefer the words "improved, but not completely successful."

I called and cancelled the bimax surgery. I then called my ENT surgeon and rescheduled the tracheostomy (the profession's "gold standard" for getting rid of OSA).

The Last Resort and Cure

The tracheostomy was easier than I expected. First, a skilled surgeon did it. He had done an average of two so-called permanent skin-lined tracheostomies per month for the previous sixteen years with no major complications. Second, I have a skinny neck and am in good health except for a mild sensory neuropathy (not counting the symptoms I have described since this mess started).

Actually, the so-called permanent tracheostomy is reversible if desired, whereas (with a few exceptions) the other two dozen or more surgeries for OSA are irreversible.

I wish I had my soft palate and uvula back (forget eating peanuts; they get stuck on the backside of what's left of my soft palate, but thankfully, no fluids come back through the nose, which some patients experience). And give back my hyoid muscle attachment (what an aggravation that has been; saliva sits and thickens in the back of my throat, causing coughing and repeated attempts to clear my throat, especially at night when lying on my back trying to doze off to sleep). By the way, I will admit, my nose is straighter after the two rhinoplasties, but do I breathe any better through my nose than before? No, not much (if at all). I look prettier, though.

I healed up in six weeks following the tracheostomy and have been free of that "Mack truck" feeling ever since. I even got some of my brain back (some will question that).

What a trip! Now we are talking four years or twenty-seven to forty-seven obstructions per hour, times eight hours, times 365 days, for four years = an estimated 315,360 to 548,960 obstructions during this journey. I ask you, does that seem like a lot of apneas to you? Well, it does to me, too.

Lessons Learned

In an ideal world, I would have been diagnosed much earlier in life, possibly as far back as my early childhood. I've had migraines (a recently recognized risk in children and teens with OSA) since I was nine years old and finally "outgrew" them in my mid-fifties. A multitude of symptoms could easily be ignored or attributed to something else, because I was not aware of what was going on in my sleep all those years (possibly my entire life, who knows?).

I wouldn't be surprised if OSA was a cause of my migraines, a recognized association, not to mention many other symptoms that came and went without explanation. All those obstructive apneas, over the years, finally and suddenly caught up with me with symptoms of severe insomnia and profound fatigue. Once heroic efforts at trying the various PAP machines failed, I would have bypassed the mandibular advancement device and all those surgeries and gone straight to a tracheostomy, avoiding four years of apneas.

I would not have wasted precious time with those futile surgeries while my body continued to be blasted repeatedly night after night from continued obstructions. Where was the urgency? There was none, not even by many sleep medicine doctors. Yet there should be the highest urgency and for some patients in dire straits, you can argue, even an emergency.

I have mentioned that the number of obstructions may vary considerably. It is a dynamic process, and the degree of airway opening depends on positioning of the body, head, and neck from minute to minute, hour to hour. A cold or flu with nasal congestion can make it worse. Weight loss or gain will change it for better or worse. Aging itself can make it worse simply from loss of tissue and muscle tone.

See the loose, sagging skin and muscles under your chin? Well, tissue in the back of the throat is loose and sagging in a similar fashion. That flabby tissue vigorously vibrating with each snore is inhaled into the tiny airway so often that the tissue itself is thought to be injured from repeated trauma, progressively worsening the problem.

One eye-opening study looked at a group of men who had so-called normal AHIs of less than 5 (AHI of 4 or less); they had repeated PSGs in six months, and nearly all of them had abnormal AHIs. Can you trust an AHI from a single PSG? The answer is no. The apneas are so variable in some patients that a single sleep test can sometimes be very misleading. Your AHI is not chiseled in stone; it is written on shifting sand and is subject to change.

Another point is that the length of each apnea and the declines in blood oxygen fluctuate. The longer the apneas or the lower the blood oxygen levels, the greater the risk. Alcohol, sedatives, sleeping pills, and other medications can dangerously prolong apneas and lower blood oxygen to the point of potential cardiac arrest. That is why a doctor should never prescribe a sleeping pill without knowing the patient's sleep status, a major reason a sleep test (PSG or HT) should be a routine part of a general physical exam. It is not practical yet because of the expense, but I am confident that advances in technology soon will make this possible.

We are all aware of the obesity epidemic. Well, I have news for you: Along with the obesity epidemic goes the sleep apnea epidemic (or more appropriately, "pandemic"). Is obesity causing OSA or is OSA causing obesity? The answer is, both. I will explain in a moment.

I agree with those specialists in sleep disorders medicine who believe that there is an unrecognized or unappreciated epidemic of obstructive sleep apnea in the United States, and this can, in large part, be accounted for by the obesity epidemic. With weight gain, soft tissue and fat progressively narrow the airway, which increases the risk of apnea.

It is well documented that the risk of OSA increases dramatically with weight gain. With weight loss, OSA may significantly improve or even vanish, but you cannot depend on it, and there is no way, yet, to tell in advance who will benefit.

Everybody talks about how obesity causes OSA. But little is said about how OSA causes obesity. Each airway obstruction during sleep results in a stress response within the sympathetic nervous system. The result is an outpouring of stress hormones from the adrenal glands. Cortisol is one of those hormones known to stimulate the appetite, causing uncontrollable weight gain.

Do the math. At thirty obstructions per hour, for eight hours of sleep, that is 240 surges of cortisol and of other weight-promoting hormones per night, or 87,600 a year. There are some victims who obstruct 60 or even greater than a hundred times per hour—that's 292,000 times per year! At that rate, a person could get as big as a house. Well, guess what? Some do! (Note: 77 percent of obese people and 95-plus percent of super obese people have OSA.)

Is it that obesity causes OSA or that OSA causes obesity? For those who no longer have OSA after losing those excess pounds, the obesity appears to have caused their OSA. For those who successfully lose weight, but still have OSA, it's likely that OSA caused the obesity. The important point is to lose weight. Even if OSA persists after successfully losing weight, it is not as severe and should be easier to treat with the PAP machine.

The sad fact is that a few obese apneics will continue their PAP machine use, not realizing that had they lost enough weight; they could have "cured" their OSA and no longer need a PAP machine.

Loud snoring, which so often accompanies OSA, is frequently treated lightly as a joke, passed off as a nuisance, or avoided by going to another room, getting a divorce, or being forced to resign from the hunting club. Even when the snorer is noted to stop breathing or struggle getting his/her breath, it is not taken seriously (i.e., seriously enough to prompt medical attention). The exceptions are heartening. Concerned wives who insist that a doctor see their husbands after being witness to snoring and frequent obstructions have saved many men from the Pandora's box of surprises awaiting them down the road. Men are less likely to show the same degree of concern or at least act on it. That is the way it is.

A common and surprising story is the husband who says to his worried wife, who has been concerned about his snoring and his frequent apneas, "There is nothing wrong with me. I feel fine and I don't need to go to a doctor."

I recall two examples of nurses who videotaped their husband's disturbed sleep and showed it to them the next day. Both saw their physicians posthaste, had PSGs documenting the disorder, and did well on CPAP. Both commented later that they could not believe how much more alert and energetic they were, whereas before, they were convinced that there was nothing wrong. They apparently developed a tolerance for feeling lousy or at least functioning at a lower level without realizing it.

One middle-aged man finally gave in to his wife's pleading, and, after successful PAP treatment, said essentially the same thing and added, "You know what? I don't have atrial fibrillation anymore!"

What is so frustrating is that no one seems to take OSA seriously (the exception being the worried wife). Is it simply a matter of the word not getting out? Or is the concept just too simple to believe or too complex to comprehend? I do suspect, sadly, that aside from the level of health education being abysmally low in this country, some apneics' brains may be too addled to get the message. They simply refuse to be bothered by such "hogwash" and eventually slip into a demented state or some other complication without ever having the benefit of treatment.

Some physicians outside the field of sleep medicine have not gotten the message yet either. I could go on about the shortcomings of medicine and the lack of sleep education in medical schools, but that subject would require another book.

Suffice it to say, your doctor may not know much about OSA for various reasons (there are exceptions, of course), so it is up to you to learn as much as you can. Unfortunately, there are not enough sleep specialists, and there never will be at the rate they are entering the field. The answer is that all physicians—not just sleep medicine specialists—should be involved in the diagnosis and treatment of OSA as it applies to their own specialty. What medical specialty is not affected by OSA? There is none.

You do not have to have a disease of nerve (neuropathy), muscle (myopathy), or a combination (neuromyopathy) to explain the epidemic of OSA, but there very well may be some as-yet-undetermined neurological disorder responsible. There are some reports that there is some neuropathology of the upper airway playing a role, but the details are yet to be worked out.

Is there something else contributing to the loss of tissue and muscle tone? Could it be that OSA itself speeds or enhances the aging process? I believe so. Obviously, age, with the loss of tissue and muscle tone, plays a major role, as does obesity. Not surprisingly, OSA risk increases with obesity even at a very young age.

And how about the study showing 75 percent of one hundred

retired NFL linemen had severe OSA[17]—and that commercial truck drivers have a risk that is similar to NFL linemen. I understand that state governments are taking on the issue, but to what degree of success, I do not know. Meanwhile, I will keep a healthy distance from all eighteen-wheelers when driving.

OSA has probably existed since humans drew their first breath. Go back through history and check out some of the possibilities. Which of the famous and infamous were likely to have suffered from OSA? Start with the big and older men and women to make it easy. The historians could have a field day. That raises the question, "What influence has OSA had on history?"

Now, look around. You can spot some casualties of OSA at a distance. Start with the older man or woman who is overweight or obese. It is the man with the seventeen-inch neck and the woman with the sixteen-inch neck who are at a higher risk. The guys with the big bellies are a sure bet. How many celebrities, congressional representatives, governmental officials, and famous personalities qualify? Potentially, quite a few. The sad fact is that most of them haven't the slightest idea that OSA may be haunting them nightly while asleep.

Struggling with their obesity are some well-known radio show and TV personalities who haven't a clue that OSA is the likely culprit. PAP treatment frequently results in weight reduction without even trying. But getting this message to them is next to impossible.

Tim Russert comes to mind. Tim had the profile (obesity with recent weight gain, high blood pressure, and blood sugar in the pre-diabetic range) for OSA. In my opinion, it is very likely that he had the disorder based on what we know now. If his wife or family noted his snoring and pauses (apneas), then he had it. Was he tested for it? Was he on a PAP machine and did he use it faithfully? We will probably never have answers to these questions. I mentioned this on an Internet blog with a group of cardiologists, and they thought my ideas were absurd.

I have heard more recently that the cardiologists are beginning to get the message about sleep apnea, though.

Is it possible had Tim Russert been on a PAP machine, using it faithfully, he might well be alive today? Yes, it is possible, if he had OSA, but we will never know.

I am concerned that the former vice president, Dick Cheney, may have OSA. He has the perfect profile. He is the right age, overweight, with coronary artery disease and atrial fibrillation requiring cardioversion on at least two occasions. We have seen him dozing at conferences more than once on television. The description given by his family in *Time* magazine was classic for the disorder. I e-mailed the White House with a message of my concern, assuming that his physicians were well aware of his sleep status, but realizing that all too frequently, attending physicians haven't a clue. I got no response and realistically did not expect one. The fact that he required another cardioversion gives me reason to doubt that he has been treated for OSA, but then again, I could be wrong.

I cannot dismiss the thought that former President Reagan may have had it and went undiagnosed and untreated, as did Charlton Heston and Rita Hayworth. Does Margaret Thatcher have it? Surely, her physicians are the best in the country, and this question has been dealt with long ago, but I am doubtful.

What about Michael Jackson; did he have sleep apnea? What little we know at the time his doctor found him in bed not breathing and with a weak pulse certainly raises the question. Giving him medications for anxiety, sleeping pills and narcotics could have been his undoing.

Let us not forget, you can be slim and trim and have severe sleep apnea. It is usually because of a small lower jaw and a receding chin (either something from birth or a family trait). A neurologist sleep specialist friend of mine told me some years ago that the worst case of

OSA that he had seen in his twenty years of sleep medicine practice was in a twenty-seven-year-old woman who stood five foot, seven inches and weighed 118 pounds. While asleep, she was blocking her airway over a hundred times per hour. Conclusion: Severe OSA can occur in someone you would least expect.

Everyone should have a sleep test. I once, half jokingly, said to some of my associates at a sleep seminar that everyone has OSA until proven otherwise. Now I am dead serious. How do you know whether you have it or not? You do not. You could have it and feel perfectly fine for years.

What is the answer? Everyone should be tested whether you are symptomatic or not; fat or not; old or not. Moreover, you should be checked periodically, like every two to five years (this frequency still needs to be explored), or more often if necessary. A sleep check should be part of a routine medical examination. I predict that it will be, once the cost is affordable. How about a home test for $50 or less? Pick it up at Wal-Mart or CVS and bring it in to have it downloaded in the physician's office on the day of your exam (dream on).

Until then, when I say tested, I mean have a polysomnogram or home test done, either by a certified or accredited sleep lab or by a certified tech under the direction of a board-certified sleep specialist. Even then, you can have a bad test (i.e., you can be misdiagnosed as "normal sleep" or "no evidence of sleep apnea" when you actually did not sleep).

A recent study showed that some patients with symptoms of OSA who had an AHI of less than 5 (considered "normal" or "acceptable") on a first test were retested later and found to have AHIs of greater than 5 ("abnormal"). Just another good reason for routine testing at regular intervals when it becomes practical.

The irony is that sometimes the diagnosis of OSA is already made by the observant spouse (at no cost except lost sleep) before the patient is even seen by the sleep specialist. My daughter diagnosed it in two friends. A mother and father, just down the street, diagnosed it in their son. My mother diagnosed it in my father. Most of us have seen or heard someone snoring and stop breathing. Diagnosis: sleep apnea.

An increasing number of sleep studies are being done at home (likely the wave of the future). I believe this is a good move, particularly in terms of cost savings, and the patient is much more likely to sleep comfortably in his or her own bed.

There is the potential for considerable savings with HT, costing in the range of a tenth or less of a PSG. To date, only Medicare has approved payment for HT. You can bet that most if not all health insurance companies will be on board before long.

Just make sure you are not sent home without the tech being informed if you are unable to sleep throughout the night. This happened to me twice and I did not have enough sense to speak up. I attribute that, in part, to an OSA befuddled brain. These studies should be repeated at no additional cost using a sleeping pill if necessary (under controlled conditions, it is safe; otherwise, never take a sleeping pill at home if you have untreated sleep apnea).

I have heard of more than one case of a wife who finally got her husband to go get a PSG, and he returned home with a "normal" test. The husband still snored and stopped breathing frequently throughout the night. He complained, "I just could not sleep in that lab." I advised one wife to have her husband go back to the lab and tell them I sent them for another study at no cost because he had "first-night effect" and did not have an adequate test. I told them to ask if it would be permissible (from the physician in charge, of course) to take a sleeping pill to make sure he got a reliable test. A well-trained tech will not make this mistake. Some labs give a sleeping pill routinely to eliminate the problem of "first-night effect." Other labs prefer the patient as is (i.e., without the use of sleeping pills), fearing that the PSG will be "contaminated." I prefer a sleeping pill to almost guarantee a good sleep test for PSGs.

I do not want to confuse the issue, but there is a condition called "sleep misperception" where the patient believes he or she did not sleep a wink or did not sleep very well, but actually slept reasonably well as evidenced by the various sleep stages that are clearly on the recording. There should be no confusion between the two states in an accredited sleep disorders lab.

There is another nagging question that has slowly dawned on me (remember, I am a recovering sleep apneic). My original symptoms of insomnia and profound fatigue were of *sudden onset,* at three a.m. one morning and did not change significantly (except for one unexplained three-day period) until four years later, several months after the tracheostomy was performed. The symptoms did not come on gradually or slowly over a prolonged period, they were abrupt. In neurology, when symptoms or signs come on suddenly, we think "stroke syndrome" meaning that there is a strong possibility of a blockage of an artery or arteries shutting off the blood flow to a part of the brain. That is, the sudden onset of a neurological deficit (like a paralysis of an arm and leg or loss of speech or sudden blindness in one eye) or even the symptoms I experienced, have that characteristic of suddenness, implying that I may have had something equivalent to a stroke. After viewing the DTI scans of the forty-one OSA patients described previously, this possibility appears more likely. Could one of those areas of damage similar to those seen on the MRI-DTI scans have been responsible for my symptoms?

Why am I telling you all this? Here is why. I tried every PAP machine available and none gave me the slightest improvement of my symptoms. This was before the "smart cards" became available. Today's PAP machines have the capability of recording a night's sleep on a microprocessor which can be removed and downloaded on a computer the next day. The number of apneas and the air pressures needed to overcome them are displayed in graphic form. From this information one can determine whether the machine is actually doing what it is supposed to do. But back in my day, eight years ago, we had no smart cards. It was assumed that since my symptoms did not improve, the machine failed to keep my airway open. I kept complaining that I was no better. If I had been able to access a smart card, I may have found that the machine was working perfectly and the reason my symptoms were not improving was from another cause. For example, suppose that I actually had one of those "MRI-DTI-like" strokes. My symptoms would not be expected to improve after one night on a PAP machine. Strokes may take weeks, months, or years to improve. (A likely explanation in my case, but I have no MRI-DTI scan to prove it).

What am I saying? Just because your symptoms do not improve after one night or a week or more on a PAP machine, does not mean the machine is not working properly. Today you do not have to guess how well your machine is functioning. It all can be recorded within the machine itself for you and your doctor to review any time a question arises as to how effective it is.

The machine may be functioning perfectly, but your 'brain lesions' will take time to heal. It is the sleep doctor's responsibility to determine whether your machine it keeping your airway open or not. If it is proven that it is indeed keeping your airway open throughout the night, then you must stick with the machine and wait for your brain to heal. Symptoms may not go away immediately. The presumption is that with treatment, it will take weeks, months or even years for certain types of brain damage to improve. How many patients give up their PAP machines too soon because symptoms did not improve right away?

Chapter 5. ━━━━━━
What Can You Do?

First, one must make the diagnosis of OSA. Once your sleep test (PSG/HT) is done, the medical diagnosis is in the hands of your sleep specialist after. Of course, the simplest, nonprofessional way to diagnose OSA is to have your spouse or significant other check you when you sleep. Next to an eyewitness, the use of a tape recorder is probably the cheapest and easiest method for determining sleep apnea (it will not work unless the patient snores). I mentioned the two wives who used a video camera on a tripod to record their husbands' apneas. Both husbands made appointments to see a sleep doctor immediately after watching the video of themselves struggle to breathe.

Nothing like a video to put things into perspective.

Snoring makes it easy to tell if there is an interruption in breathing or an obstruction. Listen for a few minutes, or however long it takes to detect a few apneas, and go back to sleep. You do not have to stay up all night, just long enough to document the fact that obstructions are occurring.

Some patients do not have apneas until the latter half of the night, when more rapid eye movement (REM) sleep occurs. All voluntary muscles are inactive except the diaphragm and eye muscles during REM sleep, increasing the chance for obstructions in most cases (and especially if lying on your back when the tongue is more likely to fall to the back of the throat). If you have witnessed apneas, you have made the diagnosis of sleep apnea. That is it. Now, give this information to your spouse's sleep doctor and he or she will take it from there.

Some patients have been diagnosed sitting in a chair at meetings or at the movies. Recently, I witnessed two patients doze off, snore and stop breathing while sitting in a doctor's waiting room. Diagnosis: OSA.

Suppose your partner doesn't hear any snoring and doesn't notice any apneas. Does that mean you don't have SA? The answer is, no, absolutely not. You could be one of the 20 percent of OSA patients who don't snore, making it much more difficult to recognize apneas. If you don't have a witness to your snoring with apneas, the only way to know whether you have OSA is by having a sleep test (PSG/HT), and unfortunately, even then the lab will occasionally miss the diagnosis. That's a little-known, but disconcerting, fact that must be kept in mind. If possible, I'd have a repeat test or have one done at another lab if there is any question about the validity of the sleep study.

You could make the argument that now is the time to buy a PAP machine on the Internet and start using it. My daughter has a friend who did just that and is apparently doing well. His wife diagnosed him. He is in his sixties and weighed over 300 pounds. He is now below 200 pounds and says he is a "new man."

It sounds like a great idea, but there are numerous pitfalls with that approach, and I would not recommend it. First, there are some contraindications to the use of a PAP machine like vomiting; a chronic sinus or middle ear infection; a recent head injury; an underlying lung disorder; recent ear, nose, throat, or head surgery; a stroke of certain types; or seizures, for example.

Second, there may be other problems that could be playing a role that you do not know about. For example, do you have hypothyroidism? Is there a problem in the airway like a mass or growth that should be removed? What about a neuromuscular disease, central sleep apnea (CSA), complex sleep apnea syndrome (CSAS), and so on?

Third, getting the right fit with the right mask can be a big problem with some patients. Who is going to help you resolve these problems? Having a medical or engineering background may help, but many potential issues can be difficult to resolve even in the best hands.

No matter how it is done, your doctor, a board-certified sleep specialist, or primary care physician working with a sleep specialist should be part of the process to help avoid those pitfalls and get the best treatment possible. This is your life we are talking about here. We should take it seriously.

But what if someone says, "We don't have any health insurance. My husband has lost his job and we simply can't afford the cost of a sleep evaluation, an expensive in-lab sleep test, and the price of an APAP machine. He snores and stops breathing throughout the night. He has a hard time staying awake during the day. We know he has sleep apnea. Isn't there a cheaper way for him to get treatment?"

Yes, you could skip the sleep test, because you already know he has sleep apnea. Buy an APAP machine with a smart card from the Internet and start using it right away. You will have to buy the software to download the night's recording from the smart card and learn how to interpret the display to be certain the machine functioning successfully. But you will be taking some risk as I mentioned above. Some of these risks can be ruled out simply by using common sense; others are impossible to exclude without professional help. Some would argue that if you weigh the risk of not treating OSA *vs.* the risk of treating in the face of an unknown contraindication, you are better off treating OSA and taking the risk. If it boils down to treatment *vs.* no treatment, then treatment is the better choice. Glaring exceptions are in people who are obviously seriously ill with heart, lung, neurological or other debilitating diseases that must be medically addressed while evaluating their sleep status.

APAP Machine May Be a Better Choice

If you have OSA, and your CPAP machine requires frequent titrations (pressure adjustments during a PSG in the sleep lab), then the APAP machine in my opinion, is a better choice. Some patients with complex lung or heart problems may still require CPAP. APAP is also known as an Auto PAP, or autotitrating PAP, because it has a computer chip programmed to determine the correct pressure needed to maintain an open airway breath by breath. Think of it as a variable-pressure self-adjusting machine. It is like having a "CPAP titration" with each breath free rather than the usual way CPAP titrations are done: once every three to six months in the sleep lab, at the cost of a PSG.

While you are waiting for your CPAP titration, there is a possibility that your CPAP machine is no longer working properly (i.e., no longer opening your airway), and you may be having apneas all the while. I call this the "CPAP trap," and it is potentially very bad for the patient. In its time, the CPAP machine was the best thing going and still is, for many patients, but now, with newer technology (e.g., APAP and VPAP), there are better options. There are exceptions where complex heart or lung problems may still require CPAP. There is the occasional problem with APAP in which a poorly fitting mask will leak air and the computer chip continues to increase the airflow, searching for the correct pressure. The result is a patient waking up with a high level of airflow blowing on the face. A better fitting mask can overcome this.

The new smart cards are making it easier to check the effectiveness of the machine. After a night's sleep, the card can be removed and downloaded on a computer displaying the entire night in graphic form. Some patients are buying the software and checking out their sleep status themselves. Instead of bringing the card to the sleep specialist's office for downloading, some sleep labs have the capability of monitoring the patients recorded sleep by telemetry and making recommendations by phone. (This technology was not available to me eight years ago).

BiPAP

BiPAP is bi-level positive airway pressure, where there are two levels of airflow: one for inhalation and another slightly lower pressure (by about 2 to 4 cm H_2O) to make it easier to exhale. Most machines should have bi-level capability. For me, it was an aggravation, passively trying to exhale against a forceful pressure of air that resisted my efforts. Potentially, it is another cause of disrupted sleep. For many patients, when bi-level is combined with APAP, it is a good thing.

VPAP

VPAP is a ventilator-assisted machine or backup for those patients who have central sleep apnea or complex sleep apnea syndrome, where the nerve cells in the brain stem sometimes fail to trigger a breath. The neurons are said to be "destabilized," possibly, in part, by all those repeated high blood CO2 levels throughout the years. Fortunately, it is not as common a problem as is OSA, and thanks to the PSG, it can be detected and treated with the newer VPAP machines. The ventilator backup is programmed automatically to trigger a breath when the brain stem neurons fail to do so.

Heated Humidifier

Humidified air is preferred over dry non-humidified air. At first, I didn't think I needed it, but changed my mind after trying it. Frankly, I think everyone would sleep more comfortably with it and recommend including it when purchasing a PAP machine.

Weight Loss: An Absolute Must

Obesity is a cause or major contributor to sleep apnea. But to make matters worse, OSA causes obesity—a vicious cycle that can be stopped only by maintaining an open airway with PAP when asleep and committing one's self to a weight loss plan.

Fat pads within the sidewalls narrow the upper airway. They grow larger with weight gain and severely narrow the airway opening to only a few millimeters wide. The narrower the airway, the greater the obstructions or apneas. This results in more cortisol surges driving weight gain.

Fat loss reduces the size of the fat pads, opens the airway, and reduces the number of obstructions. Weight tends to drop sometimes without even trying if the airway remains open. A few years ago, Duke University reported a study of eight morbidly obese (BMIs of over forty) patients with OSA who underwent gastric bypass surgery and lost a hundred pounds or more. Seven of the eight had a dramatic improvement in their OSA following the weight loss. There is clearly a place for gastric surgery in OSA patients who are morbidly obese.

There are a couple of cautions here. First, successful weight loss is a slow process no matter how it is done, measured in months and years. OSA must be treated with PAP during this time and, as long as it exists, probably for the rest of your life. That is right, it is a lifetime disorder unless you are one of the lucky few who can actually cure it by losing weight and keeping it off.

Obviously, a dedicated sleep time (seven to eight hours on PAP) and exercise program are as important as your dietary plan (which usually means portion control) for weight loss. Putting sleep time, exercise, and diet on automatic (allowing no exceptions) will make it easier to lose those excess pounds.

Having Surgery? S-T-O-P and Take This Test First

An estimated 80 percent of men and more than 90 percent of women with moderate or severe sleep apnea are undiagnosed.

Undiagnosed obstructive sleep apnea puts patients at risk of complications when undergoing surgery and anesthesia, especially after surgery in the recovery room. However, a few simple questions can determine if a person may have OSA and give them an opportunity to be treated for the condition before going under the knife, according to a new study in the journal Anesthesiology[18].

A new tool called S-T-O-P consists of the following four questions:

S: Do you snore loudly?

T: Do you often feel tired, fatigued, or sleepy during the daytime?

O: Has anyone observed you stop breathing during sleep?

P: Do you have or are you being treated for high blood pressure? (I would add diabetes here too.)

Answering "yes" to one or more of the questions should trigger an evaluation for OSA prior to surgery. (A "yes" to the "O" question is diagnostic of OSA, in my opinion.) "Identifying patients with OSA is the first step in preventing postoperative complications. Untreated OSA patients are known to have a higher incidence of difficult intubation, postoperative complications, increased intensive care admissions, and greater duration of hospital stay," Dr. Francis Chung, of the University of Toronto, said in a prepared statement.

The National Sleep Foundation (NSF) urges all sleep apnea patients and those who may be at risk for sleep apnea to discuss their symptoms with their doctors before undergoing any surgical procedure.

When All Else Fails

In many publications on OSA, tracheostomy is often mentioned in the last paragraph as a treatment of last resort and only in the most extreme or life-threatening circumstances. Well, I've got news for you. PAP machine-resistant OSA is an extreme or life-threatening circumstance. When all the machines and weight loss fail to keep the airway open while asleep, you are in an extreme or life-threatening condition.

When the grizzly chases you to the edge of a cliff, you have no choice: you have to go for it. But for me, the tracheostomy was a blessing, a life-saving procedure. I looked forward to getting my life back. It was my best chance to overcome OSA completely.

The surgery was uneventful. The surgeon lived up to his reputation. I cannot say as much for the post-op care, though. The nursing staff paid no attention to my fluid output and let my bladder overfill, forcing me to wear an indwelling catheter at home for over a week.

My urologist tells me this is an all-too-common problem these days. I'm telling you this, so you won't let it happen to you or your loved ones if there is a need for an in-hospital surgical procedure requiring a postoperative indwelling catheter.

Once the dime-sized hole in my trachea was fully healed in about six weeks, it was a matter of plugging the tube or stent during the day and unplugging it at night. The stent or small tube inserted in the opening (without it, the skin and soft tissue would slowly, over time, narrow the opening) is removed at night, cleaned with peroxide and again the next morning after a good night's sleep. I actually use two stents: one is an inch long and has a permanent plug for daytime use, and I use an open stent just for sleep. The daytime stent protrudes about a quarter of an inch and is non-obtrusive. The end is the size of a dime. It is not visible wearing a mock turtleneck shirt.

When taking a shower, a gentle blowing outward against the stent will prevent water from getting into the tracheostomy opening. During the day, I often forget I have a stent unless I'm reminded, rarely, by the sound of a slight air leak around the stent when talking. A small stent adjustment gets rid of it.

My only regret is that I cannot go sailing, swimming, or scuba diving anymore without taking the risk of a serious lung infection. Even though I have been an excellent swimmer all my life, an accidental plunge into the water with a tracheostomy could potentially be fatal. It's not the threat of drowning, which I think would be unlikely in my case, but it's the risk of a bacterial pneumonia as a result of infecting my lungs with dirty water that is the biggest threat. Unfortunately, the trach stent is not watertight. I am still working on that one.

It is interesting that at this stage, even though all else has failed, some still find the idea abhorrent: living with a tracheostomy. My response is, at this stage you have two choices: OSA or no OSA. Or, as the Indian chief said in the movie *Little Big Man*, "It is either life or death. Let it be life."

Chapter 6. ————
Summary

SLEEP APNEA IS KILLING us. It is part of the obesity epidemic in this country, and it is getting worse every year. In spite of the fact that the diagnosis and treatment are fairly straightforward, most individuals have either no knowledge or a very limited knowledge of the disorder and its destructive effects. In spite of the educational efforts by specialists in the field of sleep medicine and organizations like the National Sleep Foundation, the medical community has been slow to recognize the serious threat that this disorder poses.

In addition to the recognized association with obesity, diabetes, high blood pressure, heart disease, and stroke, I suspect that OSA plays a major role in either causing or initiating one or more of the diseases or disorders listed in Table 2, Chapter 2. At the very least, OSA must make these and other preexisting diseases worse and more difficult to treat.

This theory does not seem quite as implausible after viewing multiple white matter strokes in the MRI-DTI brain scans of a group of middle-aged men and women with untreated OSA. The truth will be known when more sleep studies and MRI-DTI scans are performed in larger patient populations. Yet to be determined are correlations of the specific functional losses resulting from these areas of brain damage in individual cases. DTI imaging of other groups of OSA patients is expected to be even more enlightening.

Regardless of whether these hypotheses eventually prove to be correct or otherwise, OSA remains a deadly disorder and must be treated.

My hypothesis that long-standing undiagnosed OSA is the cause of Alzheimer's disease (and one or more other dementias) can be determined with appropriate long-term studies. Supportive evidence is already beginning to accumulate. Eliminate OSA and prevent Alzheimer's disease: It could be that simple.

It may not be too late for the Alzheimer's patient to benefit from PAP treatment. Recent studies showed CPAP-treated Alzheimer's patients experienced improved sleep, quality of life, reduced daytime sleepiness and improved cognition by increasing total sleep time. Obviously, it would be a monumental task to treat large numbers of AD patients with PAP machines or tracheostomies, but with the prospect of improving or reversing the disorder, the idea of more intensive long treatment should be given serious consideration.

An inexpensive, foolproof home sleep test (HT) should be done on everyone and become part of the health record, just as blood pressure, pulse, and respirations are part of the routine examination. This may sound a bit much to some doctors, I know, but with a little tweaking of the current technology, I believe it will eventually happen.

Having surgery? Do not forget the STOP test. It could save your life.

Finally, of all the PAP machines, the APAP with a smart card, in my opinion, is the machine of choice, for most, to best control OSA. In that rare patient in which an all-out attack of intensive treatment with the PAP machine and weight loss fails, then the question arises: Is there an ENT surgical procedure that can convert me from a PAP machine failure to a PAP machine success? If not, then the "the gold standard," a tracheostomy, is the ultimate treatment for a life-saving cure.

Until obstructive sleep apnea is fully appreciated by both the general public and the entire medical community, millions of its victims worldwide, unaware of their plight, will continue to suffer its disastrous consequences. Isn't it time we woke up to the reality of this deadly sleep disorder and put an end to it?

Abbreviations

AASM: American Academy of Sleep Medicine.

AD: Alzheimer's disease.

AHI: apnea-hypopnea index, the total number of apneas and hypopneas (shallow breathing) during a night's sleep divided by the number of hours of sleep.

ADD/ADHD: attention deficit disorder/attention deficit hyperactivity disorder (a T&A is the cure for many children with ADD/ADHD and OSA).

APAP: autotitrating positive airway pressure, a machine with a computer chip that automatically adjusts the pressure needed to overcome each obstruction. The PAP machine I recommend for OSA.

BiPAP: bi-level positive airway pressure (two pressure settings—one for inhalation and a slightly lower one for exhalation, making it easier to exhale).

BMI: body mass index (overweight >25–30, obese >30–40, morbidly obese >40, super obese >50). Google "BMI" and check yours.

CPAP: continuous positive airway pressure, a machine that supplies a continuous flow of room air at a predetermined pressure setting measured in centimeters of water (range: 5–20+ cm H_2O; average: 8–12 cm H_2O).

DTI: diffusion tensor imaging is an MRI-based neuroimaging technique that allows the visualization of the location, the orientation, and the anisotropy of the brain's white matter tracts.

EEG: electroencephalogram, commonly called the "brain wave test," a recording of the electrical activity of the brain.

MAD: mandibular advancement device, a custom-made mouthpiece to move the lower jaw forward.

MCI: Mild cognitive impairment, a transition stage between the thinking abilities of normal aging and the more serious problem of dementia (commonly Alzheimer's disease). It is the very earliest stage of dementia.

OSA: obstructive sleep apnea, repeated airway obstruction during sleep.

PAP: positive airway pressure, any of the machines that supply a continuous flow of room air to maintain an opening in the airway. This is a general term that includes CPAP, BiPAP, APAP, and VPAP machines.

PSG: polysomnogram—the overnight electronic recording of sleep activity in a sleep laboratory.

Pes monitor: esophageal pressure monitor, used as part of a PSG when there is a need to know if the normal negative pressure is exceeded within the chest when inhaling, a possible sign of upper airway resistance syndrome (UARS).

REM: rapid eye movement, sleep stage in which there is active dreaming and inactivity of all voluntary muscles (except the diaphragm and eye muscles). More frequent during the last half of the night.

SA: sleep apnea, absence of breathing during sleep, most often due to OSA. (Central sleep apnea and complex sleep apnea syndrome are much less common.)

T&A: tonsillectomy and adenoidectomy, surgical removal of the tonsils and adenoids.

UARS: upper airway resistance syndrome, inhaling through a very narrowed airway (like inhaling through a straw), resulting in a much greater negative pressure inside the chest than normal. A potentially serious condition in which the walls of the heart may collapse, resulting in cardiac arrest.

UPPP (UP3): uvulopalatopharyngoplasty, removal of the soft palate, uvula, tonsils, and adenoids, one of the surgeries I believe should be abandoned because it does not eliminate all apneas.

VPAP: ventilator-assisted positive airway pressure, a machine used for central sleep apnea and complex sleep apnea syndrome when the brainstem neurons fail to trigger a breath. The backup ventilator will automatically breathe for you when the brainstem neurons fail to do so.

Terminology ——————————————————

Alpha waves: one type of brain wave commonly detected by electroencephalogram (EEG) in the frequency range of 8 to 12 Hz (cycles per second) and originates in the occipital lobes in the back of the brain during periods of waking/relaxation with the eyes closed. Conversely, alpha waves are low in amplitude with open eyes and during drowsiness and light sleep.

Apnea: temporary cessation of breathing, from Greek, meaning "breathless."

Apneic: one who has apnea.

Bimax: short for maxillomandibular advancement surgery, a procedure where the jaw (mandible) is sawed loose and moved forward about a half inch and the upper mouth (maxilla) is sawed free and moved forward the same amount. The gaps are filled with bone grafts from the outer layer of the skull or from the pelvis. There are well-placed pins that hold things in place for six months or more until healing is complete. It is supposed to open up the upper airway to prevent OSA.

I chose to bypass the bimax because it only reduced the number of apneas, but did not eliminate all of them.

CPAP titration: a tedious procedure to determine the correct airway pressure to overcome apneas. The sleep tech adjusts the pressure remotely from an observation room during an in-lab sleep test (PSG) until a satisfactory pressure is determined.

Cognitive: relating to mental action or process of acquiring knowledge and understanding through thought, experience, and the senses.

Dementia: loss of mental functions, such as memory, thinking, and reasoning. There are many causes of dementia. Some can be reversed or cured. Alzheimer's disease, the most common of the dementias, has no known cure—yet.

Hyoid myotomy: surgical separation of the hyoid muscle (above the Adam's apple) in an effort to open the upper airway.

Hypopnea: shallow breath.

Linguoplasty: surgical removal of part of the back of the tongue.

Rhinoplasty: nose surgery, including straightening the nasal septum.

Tracheostomy: "trach" for short. Surgical opening in the trachea (windpipe) to bypass PAP-resistant obstructions in the upper airway. Called the "gold standard" (figuratively the best, the most reliable) because when all else fails, a trach has a 99.9 percent success rate (barring an unusual complication). It is referred to as a skin-lined "permanent tracheotomy" because it can be left open permanently; however, the opening can be surgically closed or reversed if desired. Take note that almost all of the ENT surgeries performed for OSA are irreversible. For example, once the soft palate and uvula are removed in a UPPP, they cannot be replaced.

Case Histories ━━━━━━━━━━━━━━━━

THE CASES DESCRIBED ARE real; however, in some instances, details regarding identities have been changed to protect the individual's privacy.

Case 1. A seven-year-old boy in the second grade, doing poorly. He was easily distracted, was hyperactive, and could not sit still. His teachers thought he had ADHD. His parents noted his snoring at night while asleep. Sometimes he would stop breathing. A friend suggested that his pediatrician see him for probable OSA and to have a tonsillectomy and adenoidectomy (T&A). After the operation, his behavior dramatically improved. He became calm, inquisitive, and sociable and is, academically, in the top of his class. His parents say he now sleeps normally (this is an example of ADHD caused by OSA and cured by T&A).

Case 2. A secretary in her thirties underwent numerous unsuccessful surgical procedures for OSA and, as a last resort, was advised to undergo a tracheostomy. She had the procedure without complications and over the next several weeks was able to sleep soundly and regain her health. After three months, however, she returned to her surgeon, begging him to reverse the procedure because she did not like the cosmetic appearance of the trach tube protruding from her neck. Her surgeon reluctantly followed her wishes and reversed the tracheostomy (closed the opening). Within three months, she returned, complaining she could not stand it any longer: OSA was destroying her. She begged to undergo the tracheostomy again (her surgeon was kind enough to refrain from telling her "I told you so."). She learned that having an opening in her trachea was better than having OSA.

Case 3. A seventy-two-year-old former college football lineman (BMI 31) with two sons in their late thirties. They, like their father, are big men. The older son stands six feet, three inches (BMI of 37). The younger son is six feet tall (BMI 32). Both have OSA and have been on CPAP for eleven years. Their father developed diabetes and had a stroke several years ago. His wife insisted he see a sleep doctor because of loud snoring and frequent gasps for breath. She believed that he had the same problem that her sons had. A friend, who had OSA himself, joined in later, and finally convinced him to see a sleep doctor. His PSG revealed an AHI of 37. On CPAP, he exclaimed, "I can't believe it, I can think more clearly, and I have more energy than I have had in years." A known heavy snorer all his adult life, he most likely had the disorder since his late twenties, which is the age his sons were when they were diagnosed. He was diagnosed by his wife but not treated until after he developed diabetes and had a stroke.

Case 4. In the early eighties, a friend and I took a weekend bus tour to Paris from Ramstein Air Force Base. We rode shotgun up front next to the driver during the overnight trip. The driver, an obese man in his sixties, kept nodding off at the wheel. My friend and I sat frozen in abject terror. His relief driver finally took over in the wee hours of the morning, none too soon. Knowing what I know now, I cannot believe I did not have enough sense to tell him, "Stop the bus, we are getting off!" We, and the other passengers, are lucky to have survived. It is a good bet that he had OSA.

Case 5. My daughter heard a girlfriend snoring and obstructing one night on a visit. She saw her primary care physician shortly thereafter. He told her to go home and lose weight. That was it! That was his treatment for OSA! This is an example of what is known as a medical informational lag or, in my book, incompetence on the part of her primary care doctor. Of course, she should lose weight, but she also should have been started on a PAP machine immediately, not sometime in the distant future when she almost certainly finds she is unable to lose weight and has possibly suffered one or more of the complications of OSA.

Case 6. A middle-aged salesman at one of the sleep meetings I attended stood about six foot, three inches and weighed 250 pounds. He said he was nagged by his wife to go get his sleep checked because he snored loudly and was heard gasping for breath. He insisted there was nothing wrong, that he felt fine. He added that his only health problem—besides being overweight—was a heart irregularity (atrial fibrillation). He reluctantly gave in and had a PSG. The test showed an AHI of 57. Now on a PAP machine with a nasal mask, he said, "I cannot believe it, I am more energetic and I can think better. I must have gotten used to feeling bad." He added, "Oh, by the way, I don't have atrial fibrillation anymore." (An example of cardiac arrhythmia caused by OSA and reversed by PAP in another patient who denied having problems, and yet another wife to the rescue.)

Case 7. A twenty-four-year-old real estate agent complained of frequently waking with a gasp from sleep, saying, "It's like I have to catch my breath." She is obese and worried about uncontrollable weight gain. She has been experiencing a lack of energy and moodiness for several months, adding, "I'm not myself." Her father has been using a PAP machine for ten years. She has come to the realization that she too may have the same problem as her father. She plans to see a sleep specialist as soon as she can get an appointment.

Case 8. A nurse insisted that her husband see his doctor because of

65

his loud snoring and apneas. He refused. She put her video camera on a tripod, took an all-night video of him sleeping, and showed it to him the next morning. He made an appointment that day. On a PAP machine, he exclaimed, "I can't believe it, I have more energy and I am able to think more clearly." Another nurse told me a similar story. (These are examples of patients again not taking the problem seriously and caring wives saving their husbands' lives with a video camera.)

Case 9. I saw an elderly man and his wife in my office. Their daughter spoke to me privately to tell me that she was visiting them from out of town and discovered they both snored loudly and had frequent apneas while asleep. Neither of her parents knew the other had a problem. They were both referred to a sleep specialist. (This is an example of how a visiting family member can come to the rescue.)

Case 10. I was exercising at a local gym when the wife of an air force pilot asked about her husband's loud snoring and long silent pauses. He sometimes woke up gasping. I urged her to have him see a sleep specialist because of the seriousness of OSA. She said she would try to get him to see a sleep specialist, but doubted that he would follow through because he would probably be grounded. I have no idea of the Air Force's policy regarding OSA, but I trust that systems are in place to effectively deal with this. (This is an example of OSA patients concealing their health status to keep their jobs at their own and possibly others' peril.)

Case 11. I met a gentleman in his seventies at a local gym recently and asked him, "Do you have sleep apnea?" I had noted his obesity and brave attempts to complete his workout, and it struck me that he had the perfect profile for OSA. "Yes, I was diagnosed in 1996 and have been on CPAP since," he said. "My daughter caught me snoring, and I stopped breathing while asleep on the couch; she made me go to the doctor. I weighed 380 pounds and after I went on CPAP, I lost 200 pounds. Two years before I went on CPAP, my doctor told my family I had Alzheimer's disease. I didn't know my own name. I am now attending college and plan to teach. I have a 4.0 average, and I am having the time of my life." Suppose his daughter had not witnessed her father's apneas. Where would he be now? Since Alzheimer's patients' life expectancy is less than ten years, he might be dead! Could this be an example of the reversal of Alzheimer's disease with CPAP therapy? I believe so. And again, a loving family member, his daughter, saved his life.

Case 12. My father snored heavily and was known to stop breathing while asleep all his adult life. OSA was confirmed by a sleep test in the mid-1980s, but he flatly refused CPAP treatment because of claustrophobia from the nasal mask. Within ten years, he was diagnosed with Alzheimer's disease. Ten years later, he died at home, of pneumonia. He was eighty-five. If my hypothesis is correct, my father had a classical case of Alzheimer's disease brought on by OSA. His father died in a nursing home with the diagnosis of dementia, most likely AD.

Appendix A. ——————
Useful Web Sites

Sleep Disorders

www.sleepeducation.com, The American Academy of Sleep Medicine (AASM) provides facts about sleep, sleep disorders, treatments, and services. Online discussion forum and latest news from the leader in sleep medicine.

www.sleepfoundation.org The National Sleep Foundation is a nonprofit organization funded largely by several pharmaceutical companies. It has been a good source of sleep disorders information.

www.nhlbi.nih.gov/about/ncsdr/, The U.S. National Center on Sleep Disorders Research of the National Institutes of Health supports sleep research, training, and education to improve health.

www.sleepapnea.org, a good source of information for the layperson.

www.webmd.com/sleep-disorders/sleep-apnea/sleep-apnea. It is always informative.

www.mayoclinic.com/health/sleep-apnea/DS00148/ A great place to find answers.

www.sleepcenters.org Go to this Web site to find doctors in your area who are experts at helping people who have sleep problems. The site has an online directory of sleep centers and labs. It has a map that enables you to search for help by state. Each center and lab in the directory meets the AASM's high standards for accreditation.

www.nhlbi.nih.gov/health/dci/Diseases/SleepApnea/SleepApnea_WhatIs.html

Animation of OSA

http://www.youtube.com/watch?v=mjQdAf9cQBo Check out some of these videos on sleep apnea. Some are difficult to watch.

Alzheimer's Disease

www.mayoclinic.com/health/alzheimers-disease/ds00161, a comprehensive overview.

www.alzheimers.org, Alzheimer's Disease Education and Referral Center.

www.alzfdn.org, Alzheimer's Foundation of America.

www.medicinenet.com/alzheimers_disease/article.htm Causes, Symptoms, Diagnosis and Treatment

For All Neurological Diseases

www.thebrainmatters.org The American Academy of Neurology (AAN) patient Web site.

www.neurologynow.com "Neurology Now: Healthy Living for Patients and Their Families" is an official publication of the AAN. (Free subscriptions are available to individuals with a neurological disorder and their caregivers/families.)

Appendix B. ———
Further Reading

Lawrence Epstein, Steven Mardon The Harvard Medical School Guide to a Good Night's Sleep (Harvard Medical School Guides) (Paperback), 2007.

Nancy Foldvary-Schaefer, Getting a Good Night's Sleep (A Cleveland Clinic Guide) (Cleveland Clinic Press) (Illustrated, paperback) May 2006.

T. Scott Johnson, William A. Broughton, and Jerry Halberstadt, Sleep Apnea: The Phantom of the Night: Overcome Sleep Apnea Syndrome and Win Your Hidden Struggle to Breathe, Sleep, and Live (New Technology Publishing) (Paperback) 2003.

Burton Abrams, The Perils of Sleep Apnea: An Undiagnosed Epidemic: A Layman's Perspective, (iUniverse) (Paperback) 2007.

Barbara Phillips and Matthew T. Naughton, Obstructive Sleep Apnea (Fast Facts) (Health Press) (Paperback) 2007.

Peretz Lavie, Restless Nights: Understanding Snoring and Sleep Apnea (Yale University Press): New Haven and London, 2003.

Author's Biography ——————

Mack D. Jones, MD, SAAN, is a board-certified clinical neurologist. A graduate of the Medical College of Georgia, he completed his neurology residency at the University of North Carolina in Chapel Hill, North Carolina. He joined the clinical staff as an assistant professor in the Department of Neurology at the Medical College of Georgia. He is now retired in Fort Walton Beach, Florida after twenty-seven years in private practice. Contact Dr. Jones by e-mail at: jonesmd3@gmail. com.

References

1   Richard B Berry, et al., Portable Monitoring and Autotitration versus Polysomnography for the Diagnosis and Treatment for Sleep Apnea (Journal of Sleep and Sleep Disorders Research), 31(10), 2008, 1423–1431.

2   Malcolm Kohler, et al. Even Mild Sleep Apnea Ups Heart Risk. (American Journal of Respiratory and Critical Care Medicine), November 1, 2008.

3   Shahar, et al. AHIs of 1–10 Are Associated with Increased Cardiovascular Risk. (American Journal of Respiratory and Critical Care Medicine), 2001.

4   Young T, et al. The Occurrence of Sleep-Disordered Breathing Among Middle-aged Adults. (The New England Journal of Medicine, 29; 328 (17); 1230–3, 1993

5   Paul M. Macey, et al. Brain Structural Changes in Obstructive Sleep Apnea. (SLEEP), 31(7), 2008, 967–977.

6   Ariel Tarasiuk, et al. The Effect of Obstructive Sleep Apnea on Morbidity

and Health Care Utilization of Middle-Aged and Older Adults (Journal of the American Geriatrics Society) 3/27/2008.

7   Miranda Hitti. Obstructive Sleep Apnea May Trigger Nighttime Heart Attacks. (Journal of the American College of Cardiology), 2008.

8   José A. Luchsinger, et al. Relation of Diabetes to Mild Cognitive Impairment. (Archives of Neurology) 64(4), 2007, 570–575.

9   Christine Reitz, et al. Hypertension and the Risk of Mild Cognitive Impairment. (Archives of Neurology). 64(12), 2007, 1734–1740.

10 Xiulian Sun, et al. Hypoxia Facilitates Alzheimer's Disease Pathogenesis by Up-Regulating BACE1 Gene Expression. PNAS (Proceedings of the National Academy of Sciences), 103(49), 2006, 18727–18732.

11 Rafesh Kumar, et al., June 27, 2008 issue of Neuroscience Letters, sleep apnea patients were found to have shrunken brain structures called "mammillary bodies" involved in memory, the University of California at Los Angeles (UCLA).

12 Adam P. Spira, et al. Disordered Breathing and Cognition in Older Women. (Journal of the American Geriatrics Society), 56(1), January 2008, 45–50.

13 Kadotani H, Association Between Apolipoprotein E epsilon4 and Sleep-Disordered Breathing in Adults. (JAMA), 2001 Sep 26; 286; (12); 1447–8.

14 Jana R. Cooke, et al. CPAP Improves Sleep in Patients with Alzheimer's Disease and Sleep-Related Breathing Disorders. American Academy of Sleep Medicine. University of California at San Diego.

15 M. S. Chung, et al. Continuous Positive Pressure Reduces Subjective Daytime Sleepiness in Patients with Mild to Moderate Alzheimer's

Disease with Sleep Disordered Breathing. (American Geriatric Society) 54(5), 2006, 777–781.

16 Jana R. Cooke, et al. CPAP Improves Sleep in Patients with Alzheimer's Disease and Sleep-Related Breathing Disorders. American Academy of Sleep Medicine. University of California at San Diego.

17 The Mayo Clinic and New York University. Linemen Have a Greater Prevalence of Obstructive Sleep Apnea (OSA). An ongoing study of a hundred retired NFL players was conducted. In the total group of players including all positions, the prevalence of OSA approximated 50 percent. In linemen, the prevalence increased to 75 percent, and the majority had a severe category of this disorder. Commercial truckers, who tend to be large men, have a somewhat similar prevalence of OSA compared to retired NFL players.

18 Frances Chung, et al. S-T-O-P. Undiagnosed Obstructive Sleep Apnea Can Be Revealed Preoperatively by a Simple Eight-item History. (Anesthesiology), May 2006.

LaVergne, TN USA
03 September 2009
156804LV00001B/57/P

9 780595 528707